Praise for
RETURN TO CENTER

"In *Return to Center*, Rocky Snyder has done it again! Providing world class functional health instruction & information in a user friendly, informative way, all the while conveying his deep knowledge and caring for his reading audience. A must-read for athletes and general population alike!"

GERARD "GP" PEARLBERG, professional running coach, USATF; author of *Run Tall, Run Easy*; head coach, Boomer Esiason Foundation NYC

"The fitness industry is currently undergoing a revolution. Going to the gym is no longer simply about getting pumped or just for looking good in the mirror. It has become a place for developing true physical fitness and restoring healthy, pain-free lifestyles. Rocky Snyder is at the forefront of this revolution, and this book provides a clear guide to discovering your individual needs for mobility and strength. It is ideal for both trainers and people who want to take charge of their physical fitness. It is packed with great storytelling, case studies, the importance of self-assessment/reassessment, and goes into great detail on how the nervous system rules the roost. Rocky has taken over 25 years of experience and has integrated the brilliance of Gary Ward's Flow Motion Model® to provide the best exercise selection for every individual, based on his/her current movement profile. I've started applying the concepts of this book to my own mobility and strength programs, and I'm noticing dramatic improvements already! Rocky's approach, clearly outlined in this book, needs to become the standard of modern-day fitness and training."

ERIC LAZAR, physical therapist, Madrid College of Chiropractic

"*Return to Center* is an essential book for understanding how to live and perform well in your body for a lifetime, whether in daily activities or high-level athletics. The soundness of the principles Rocky writes about in this book, and his skill and expertise in applying them, has made it possible for me to achieve every one of my goals as an older athlete in water polo, without injury; including two world championships and multiple national championships."

JOEL F. WADE, PH.D., author of *The Virtue of Happiness*

"Rocky Snyder's always fresh, cutting-edge approach to moving intelligently jumped off the pages and into my life and practice in this important book. This is a must-read for clinicians, coaches, elite athletes, or weekend warriors–anyone who is interested in informed, thoughtful, and actionable information about applied biomechanics for your sport or lifestyle practice of choice. It's one thing to get well, but Rocky teaches us how to stay well, prevent injury, and live an active, vibrant life. A no-brainer."

DR. HERBY BELL, professor, Clinical Education Faculty, Life Chiropractic College West

"In *Return to Center*, Rocky Snyder has done an extraordinary job of investigating and delineating the many complex variables of exercise and physical training and presenting them in an accessible and very readable way to help people move better and train intelligently. I highly recommend this book to fitness professionals as well as anyone interested in improving their health and fitness."

ROBERT E. McATEE, author of *Facilitated Stretching* and *Sports Massage for Injury Care*

"All of the motion-based elements of human health are packed into this opus for the modern mover. Rocky takes us through a historical tour of the fitness 'craze' and brings us to the present moment—from movement minefield to mind body practicality. He respectfully offers a subtle, streamlined, and manageable program that speaks to professionals, practitioners, and fitness consumers alike. Within it you'll find stories of his clients who have unraveled decades of injuries, compensations, and surgical challenges into a painless life. It's a book that validates the potential in all of us to shift our structure into a newfound sense of center."

JILL MILLER, author of *The Roll Model: A Step-by-Step Guide to Erase Pain, Improve Mobility, and Live Better in Your Body*

"Utilizing this method of training & conditioning has helped me continue to compete in several marathons and shaved fifteen minutes off of my Big Sur half marathon time to achieve a personal best! This approach allows me to pursue my passion without career-ending injuries."

KATHERINE BEIERS, Boston Marathon winner in the over 80 age category

"In this age of information overload, Return to Center offers an insightful, practical method for how to assess and address limiting factors in the body. Rocky presents clear and effective strategies for re-educating the body to move more purposefully, intelligently, and freely, returning it to its full potential.

His effective approach is backed up with scientific data and clinical case studies, making this book an inspiring resource that leads directly to practical application. Rocky's system helps identify root causes of many pain symptoms, weaknesses, and movement limitations, and provides efficient, goal-oriented programs, whether for performance, fitness, or pain relief.

If you're a health professional who works with the human body—such as a physical therapist, trainer, or strength coach—or if you just want to improve your body's ability to move, Return to Center is a must-read."

JESSICA SCHATZ, The Core Expert™, Body By Jessica®, Champion Pilates™
master pilates instructor, yoga teacher, health and wellness coach

"Rocky's journey, deep investigation, and discoveries for what's actually useful in the pursuit of health, fitness, and function is distilled down in these pages. Learn to upgrade your movement patterns and discover a new model for life-long fitness."

TOM McCOOK, founder and director, Center of Balance Master Movement Educator

"I can attest to Rocky's unbelievable understanding, of the human body. His training methods can and will help you in any arena of life. As an NHL hockey player, I used many of these principles throughout my career, which I believe helped me play 16 years and over 1,000 games. Rocky is definitely one of the Elite trainers in the field today!"

SCOTT HANNAN, NHL defenseman, San Jose Sharks

"Have you ever experienced the law of diminishing returns when it comes to working out? That's when you put more and more in to get less and less back. Maybe it's time to find a new path. So, where do you look? Do not despair...here's a book written by someone who's been there, done that, and come out the other side. Rocky Snyder is not just a really good coach and personal trainer, he can write! So, if you're ready for change, and doing the 'same old same old' just isn't happening, then check out this book."

MALCOLM BALK, author of *Master the Art of Running* and *Master the Art of Workout!*

"Rocky and I live, eat, and breathe 'movement.' Whilst our movement backgrounds and specialties differ, we share the same magnificent teachings and 'sleuthing' thought processes of Gary Ward, Chris Sritharan, and the body of work that is Anatomy in Motion™, so I was excited to read Rocky's application of gait mechanics in his mastered field, that of strength and conditioning.

Turn the pages and get excited; apply the abundant knowledge and feel change happen. Regain autonomy over your body's strength and conditioning training by following this new route, packed with signposts guiding you to your best choices and laced with fascinating, relevant stories, both current and historical; Rocky is a true exponent of his craft. Let his passion and knowledge imbue you with the confidence to help yourself."

HELEN HALL, author of *Even With Your Shoes On*

"*Return to Center* is an awakening. Unlike many strength training manuals, one does not simply learn a set of universal exercises applicable to everybody. Rather, Rocky teaches his readers how to assess their own bodies, so that they can find the exercises particular to them. As a professional handball player struggling with structural shoulder issues, Rocky's functional approach enabled me to move from a top twenty player to the number two handball player in the world. An excellent teacher, Rocky shows each of us how we can reach our postural center, thereby enabling greater strength, balance, endurance, and injury prevention. *Return to Center* increases the ease with which individuals engage in everyday activities, and immensely benefits the performance and longevity of recreational and elite athletes. This is truly a book for everybody."

EMMETT PEIXOTO, professional handball player

"Finally, a strength training book that is not focused on building a body just for looks but building a body for better function, less pain, and injury prevention. Rocky's passion and dedication to educating himself and others comes full circle in this new book. You can clearly see his years of experience and education come together in this guide on how we can create individualized strength training programs for our own needs or the needs of others. We all want to save time and money. Here is the book that will do both. Instead of guessing what our bodies need to stay functioning, or paying a professional to tell us, Rocky gives us the tools to be able to assess and then work on those specific areas. Designed for both the professional and the individual, we now have the ability to restore our own body to the balance it is seeking. We can strength train safely and with purpose. *Return to Center* provides invaluable information on how to assess your own posture and function and what you can do about it."

WENDY WILLIS, corrective movement specialist, founder of West End Fitness

To Dana, Madison, and Jack.
May you be forever free to wander, but
always return to center.

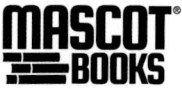

MASCOT® BOOKS

www.mascotbooks.com

Return to Center

Principal Photographer: Gary Irving www.garyfoto.com

For more information, please contact:
Mascot Books
620 Herndon Parkway #320
Herndon, VA 20170
info@mascotbooks.com

Library of Congress Control Number: 2019904414

CPSIA Code: PRV0220A
ISBN-13: 978-1-64307-548-8

Printed in the United States

RETURN TO ∞ CENTER

ROCKY SNYDER, CSCS

Strength Training to
Realign the Body, Recover from
Pain, and Achieve Optimal
Performance

TABLE OF CONTENTS

Chapter 8

THROUGHOUT THIS BOOK:

When you see a **QR code**, scan it with your phone's camera for a video tutorial of the concepts found in the book.

You are also able to go directly to my YouTube channel—Rocky Snyder, CSCS—and search for any individual exercise by name.

A NOTE FROM THE AUTHOR

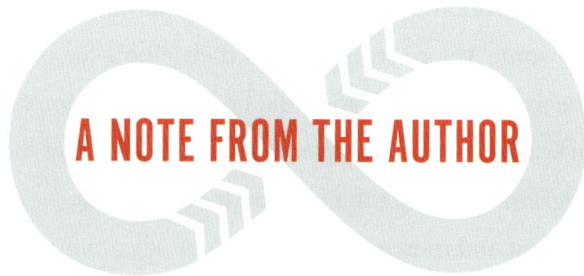

With all the machines in the health clubs, all the articles in fitness magazines, and the plethora of videos on YouTube, it is easy to be overwhelmed when figuring out how to exercise. Almost everyone begins exercising after being shown or taught by someone else, like a friend, P.E. teacher, coach, personal trainer, or a parent. Just like knowledge about culture and family traditions is passed down from generation to generation, knowledge about exercise is also passed down. What if that knowledge is incomplete or wrong?

How many people really understand the positive and negative long-term effects that traditional strength training has on their body? How many have ever asked where the exercises originated from, who created them, and why they should perform them? Or were you like me, and just took it for granted, that this is what you should do without really questioning why? It took me a very long time to ask these questions.

For many years I had this feeling that something was not quite right. If no two people were truly identical, and they moved in different ways, why would they perform precisely the same exercises? If these exercises, which are nearly universal in every gym and health club, were safe and supposed to make us stronger and more fit, why was almost everyone complaining about some painful body part? One person would complain about their knee while another spoke of rotator cuff trouble. There was always someone rubbing their lower back or shoulder, while another person wore some Velcro strap around their elbow for one reason or another. The majority of gym goers did not have such complaints before they began working out. The troubles started after they began their exercise program. Shouldn't that scream for attention?

Today, joint and muscle pain has become so common we consider it normal. If we are not in pain, then we are in between "pain periods." Even our highest-caliber athletes play in pain, or fall under the category of injured reserve. Could non-contact injuries have something to do with the conditioning exercises selected for them, and how they train their bodies?

There seems to be more orthopedic surgeons and physical therapists than ever before, with an increasing number of prescription medications, surgeries, and "syndromes." Medical corrections have become the preferred solution. Instead, what if the solution is developing a more intelligent conditioning program and improving a person's quality of movement? Some of the most common sports-related injuries are ankle sprains, pulled groins, strained hamstrings, ACL tears, shin splints, tennis elbows, golfer's elbows, and sciatica. These are all musculoskeletal problems affecting how the body moves and may be caused by the strength training exercises they are performing. Are these athletes performing the right exercises? If they are, why are they getting injured and re-injured? Could it simply be a matter of developing programs based on an individual's body and how it moves?

I am reminded of that scene in the movie *The Matrix* when Laurence Fishburne's character Morpheus, is speaking to Neo, Keanu Reeves' character. Morpheus offers two pills, a blue and a red. He tells Neo that he can take the blue pill and things will go on being the same and he can keep believing whatever he wants to believe. If he takes the red pill he will stay in Wonderland and he will be shown how far down the rabbit hole goes. This book is the red pill. Now you have a decision to make. Will you take the blue pill and stop reading here - continue going to the gym doing the workout you have always done, resulting in nagging, recurring pain and therefore avoid certain movements? Or, will you take the red pill and read on to find out what your body needs and how to create a program that will take you to the next level. Your body already knows what it needs. With the guidance of this book, you now have the ability to understand what it is telling you and free yourself from the mindset that joint pain is normal and is just a part of getting old.

The choice is yours.

Welcome to the future of fitness!

FOREWORD

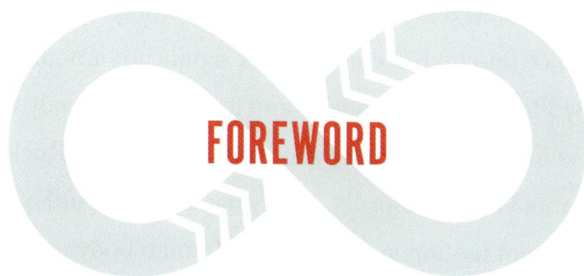

My name is Gary Ward. I began teaching my Anatomy in Motion work to share what I call the *Flow Motion Model®*. This is a discovery of how each and every joint in the human body moves in three dimensions through the walking gait cycle. The model itself guides us to not just appreciate how we walk but also how we move—in every sense of the word. The model reveals the natural movement interactions and relationships that take place in the human body. It has always been an interesting phenomenon for me that the movements we make when training or working out are often at the cost of what our bodies are truly capable of. If we are unable to access all of these natural movements in our body, what will the cost be to our bodies? Is the modern conventional way of training and exercising congruent with how our bodies need to move? Can we adjust our thinking so as to tailor our workout programs towards ensuring we can all have access to our whole joint system and be free of the shackles of movement limitation?

If there was ever a man who has committed his life to understanding movement in the realm of fitness training, it is Rocky Snyder. I had the great pleasure of meeting Rocky in 2014, in San Francisco, when I was teaching my first Anatomy in Motion Finding Centre course in the United States. Rocky very clearly had a wealth of knowledge and was intrigued by this new body of work I was presenting. We have been very close ever since and he has committed a significant amount of time to learning my Flow Motion Model® and applying it directly to his work in the fitness industry. It is enjoyed by all who frequent Rocky's Fitness Center in Santa Cruz, California. Rocky has diligently and painstakingly related every joint motion available to the human body to specific gym-based exercises that are beneficial in restoring particular movement patterns. He has presented his ideas in a very usable format, starting with how to assess a person's movements and what to consider. His work can guide you to what to do specifically for your own body. The old paradigm of fitness, strength, and conditioning is slowly changing as we move away from "strong and stable" to be more mobile and somehow, even stronger. Mobility generally seems to come down to awareness: awareness of the movements I am capable of, awareness of the movements I struggle with, awareness of how I can re-experience those movements in my body, and awareness of the changes in my body as a result of doing so. As educators we hope that people can sidestep the need to be bigger, better, faster, and stronger when it is at the cost of their own body. Rocky believes that all trainers, physical therapists, and strength coaches should all be able to help people achieve these gains, while at the same time helping them maintain their optimal and efficient movement potential. Rocky has put together this book to help you work *with* your body rather than work *on* it.

To that end, knowing what movements your body has access to and what movements it struggles with and thus does not have access to is akin to personal movement longevity. No longer need you move *around* your problems, but you can now move *with* them and *through* them until they are problems no more.

In this space, training and developing the integrity of your joint structures and your tissues using traditional movements and exercises in a more meaningful way is exactly what Rocky brings you in this book. An exercise can be more than an exercise when your intention for that exercise is to enhance the integrity of your physical system rather than just to get stronger. More mobility in your system leads to natural strength and performance gains.

If you're in the game of prescribing exercises to your clients and haven't previously considered the depths of why you prescribe that exercise (beyond aesthetic appeal and faster, stronger, bigger gains), then I am 99 percent sure you will gain value from reading this book. I invite you to diligently apply its logic to both yourself and your clients.

Gary Ward

Creator of Anatomy in Motion

Author of *What The Foot?*

@garyward_aim

@garyward_aim

BEFORE WE GET STARTED

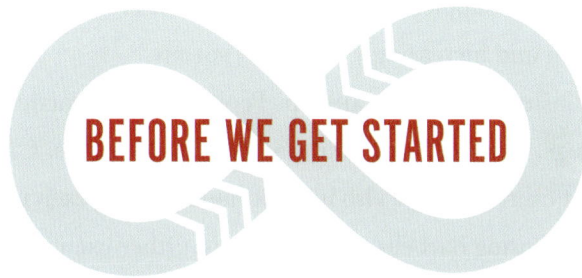

The fact that you are reading this book suggests you like moving your body and want to improve your physical performance. You might love working out, but have you ever wondered where today's strength exercises came from? How did we get to the point where we need to exercise? Why do we do the exercises we find at the gym, in the magazines, and on YouTube? In order to understand why we exercise the way we do, it is important to understand how we got here.

THE EARLY YEARS

In the mid-1800s many Americans left the family farms and headed to the urban areas. Jobs in manufacturing rose and the lure of city life drew millions to a type of lifestyle they had never experienced. For many, a full day of intense, manual labor was no longer required, and it was quickly replaced by less physical activity. Improvements in transportation and inventions of time-saving and laborsaving devices occurred at an exponential rate. As daily, purposeful physical movement diminished, and mass production of food rose, Americans began to get out of shape. Obesity had yet to reach the epidemic proportions we see today, but a need emerged for supplemental movement to offset the effects of a new, industrialized and increasingly sedentary society.

Gymnasiums began to appear. People began practicing on the moving rings, parallel bars, vault, and balance beams. Calisthenics (bodyweight exercises) were also incorporated into the exercise regimen. People started using barbells and dumbbells. Other exercise equipment

1800s gymnasium

such as climbing ropes and ladders, medicine balls, Indian clubs, and cables with weight stacks were also a regular part of gymnasiums. Strongmen traveled from town to town to thrill crowds with their amazing feats of strength. Lifting barbells, bending steel rods, and wrestling were all part of the show. One man in particular, Eugene Sandow, who is considered the "Father of Modern Bodybuilding," even wrestled a lion into submission.

Eugene Sandow

PHYSICAL EDUCATION

Public schools began to adopt European systems of exercise (Lyng and Jahn methods) to help children stay active. Physical education (P.E.) was truly about educating youth about the physical body. Unfortunately, after World War I that began to change. Somewhere between 1920 and 1930, American schools shifted the focus away from physical education and more towards sports and competition. Girls turned to field hockey, fencing, and tennis, while boys pursued football, baseball, and another emerging sport, basketball. This approach to physical education remains the same nearly 100 years later. Very little has changed. If anything, children move even less, and in many schools, physical education has become an elective. I remember when my daughter was a freshman in high school, her "final exam" for P.E. consisted of walking to the bowling alley for two games of bowling.

In the 1940s, the world was at war and the military got a first-hand understanding of the fitness level of the average citizen. Recruitment centers saw many hopeful enlistees who were overweight, out of shape, and not considered combat ready. It became apparent that, for the preservation and protection of the country, future generations needed physical fitness. After the Korean War, in 1956, President Dwight D. Eisenhower initiated the President's Council on Youth Fitness. It promoted 50-mile hikes and other military-style conditioning like that used in the Marines. For most American kids, that proved to be unpopular. President John F. Kennedy would later change the organization's name to the President's Council on Physical Fitness, but the program itself changed little. President Lyndon B. Johnson would, yet again, change the name of the program to the President's Council on Physical Fitness and Sports to encourage more sports and less education of the physical body. Johnson also implemented the President's Physical Fitness Award in 1966. The original tests were a softball throw, broad jump, 50-

yard dash, and a 600-yard walk/run. Ultimately, these tests would change as the public continued to get more de-conditioned in the ever-increasing technological world.

TV & THE SILVER SCREEN

Jack LaLanne

In 1936, the nation saw one of the first fitness gyms in Oakland, California, opened by a 21-year-old named Jack LaLanne. LaLanne would become known as the "Godfather of Fitness." He would go on to publish several books on health and nutrition, be a motivational speaker, compete in bodybuilding contests, and host his own television show from 1953 to 1985. He espoused the value of proper nutrition and full-body movement. He was one of the first trainers to challenge and encourage women and seniors to go to gyms and get exercise. Before his death in 2011, and perhaps still to this day, he proved to be an inspiration for millions. LaLanne helped open the door for other fitness enthusiasts to appear in television and movies. Perhaps this led to the birth of the action hero.

In Hollywood, during the 1950s and 1960s, there were two actors who brought strongman feats of strength and bodybuilding to the screen. Reg Park and Steve Reeves starred in roles such as Hercules and Goliath. Although most of their films were made in Italy, they became popular icons in America. These films, and Johnny Weissmuller's Tarzan films of the 1940s, inspired many to pursue bodybuilding. This included a young Austrian man by the name of Arnold Schwarzenegger.

Schwarzenegger and his fellow bodybuilders such as Lou Ferrigno, Franco Columbu, Bill Pearl, and Frank Zane, began to change the face of bodybuilding. The main goal of bodybuilding seemed to morph away from improving physical prowess to building bigger, more beautiful muscles for showing on stage and on film. Through the 1960s and 1970s, bodybuilding gained tremendous popularity; a boost came in 1977, with the film *Pumping Iron* which sent more people than ever to the gym. Although most of the exercises these people undertook involved barbells and dumbbells, there were a few other devices which began to fill up the gym rooms. Machines like the leg press, a seated device where a person drove a weighted sled up and down to increase leg strength, proved to be easier to manage and safer for the beginner to use. Plus, a person could really load up a tremendous amount of weight compared to balancing a barbell on the shoulders and squatting. As more members appeared in gyms more machines did, too. It made sense for the gym owners to reduce their liability any way they could. It was much safer to have people sitting in machines while they pushed and pulled instead of a roomful of fitness neophytes swinging dumbbells around their heads and dropping barbells at their feet. The birth of the running craze occurred in 1977 with the publication of Jim Fixx's book, *The Complete Guide to Running*. It seemed that the nation was really beginning to move.

FAST FORWARD TO TODAY

Today, it seems that exercise routines have turned into a competition. Extreme obstacle course races have become popular. A new subculture has been created. Many gyms have been influenced by such high-intensity training, and have adopted the approach and the exercises at its center. Olympic lifts, pull-ups, burpees, and box jumps are now on the menu for just about everybody. Olympic lifts, as seen in the summer Olympic games, involve pulling weights off the ground in an explosive manner and then catching the weights at shoulder height or overhead. Burpees are a sequence of movements where a person squats to the floor, lowers into a push-up, hops back to their feet before jumping off the ground and repeating. Box jumps are exactly what they sound like, jumping up on a box. The question becomes, how high? You can view plenty of "gym fails" on YouTube featuring future emergency room visitors attempting to jump up on a 36-inch-high box with large rubber weight plates stacked on top, only to fall flat on their pride.

At the same time, as cell phones continue to morph into handheld computers, and time spent on the internet is greater than ever, society's level of inactivity and obesity are reaching epidemic proportions. Americans today are more de-conditioned than any generation before them. It is the worst time to create excessively intense exercise programs for the average person. It takes most people years of poor lifestyle choices, lethargy, and overeating to create a de-conditioned body. Decreased functional capacity, combined with ultra-high levels of exercise intensity, is a foreboding combination. Applying high-intensity training to a de-conditioned body is like placing a high-performance race car engine into an AMC Pacer. Sure, it will go, but can the frame withstand all that power? Odds are, something will give. For many, the pursuit of competition makes winning more important than proper form and execution of exercises. On the upside for some, such a program means rapid weight loss and strength gains. But for many others, it means pain and lost time from enjoying other activities.

Activity Levels, Obesity Rates, and Exercise Intensity Over Time

O Activity Level   O Obesity Rate   O Exercise Intensity

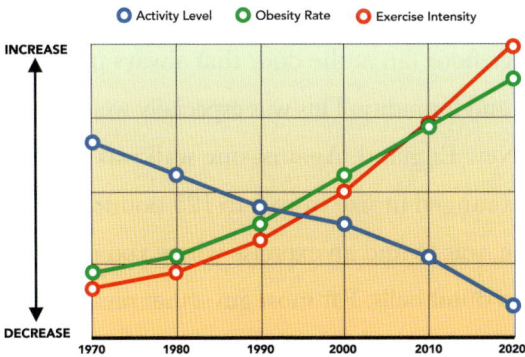

The great thing is that exercise seems to be here to stay. It is not a passing fad. It is continually changing and evolving. The question is, what is it evolving into? Will it focus primarily on aesthetics, competition, muscle size, or something else? Hopefully, the answer is that exercise programs will take into consideration several factors: improving posture, reducing pain, enhancing movement efficiency, strength, and overall body function in a world which continues to demand less movement and more deformity at younger and younger ages.

MY PATH TO PERSONAL TRAINING

I grew up in a blue-collar neighborhood in the suburbs north of Boston, playing sports and exploring the outdoors. My family did not have the extra income to spend on Pop Warner football or Little League baseball. That was fine with me, because there were plenty of kids around with whom to play street hockey, mud football, and pick-up basketball. Going to a gym to work out was not something any of us thought about. There was always so much to do right outside our front doors, we didn't need a special place to exercise. There were trees to climb, railroad tracks to hike, and marshes in which to play "Capture the Flag." It was not until my senior year in high school that I actually went to a gym.

The gym was something that resembled a cleaned-out chicken coop—and it smelled pretty similar! It was a small, rectangular building with only one door in and out. The little windows along one side could open only a few inches, just enough to circulate the smell of sweat and body odor. There was a large floor fan at the door that always pointed outward to remove the heat and humidity. This was especially welcomed in the summer months in New England. Against one wall was a long row of rusty dumbbells that ranged in size from 5 to 125 pounds. The goal, it seemed, for everyone, was to find an exercise where you needed to use the pair of 125-pound dumbbells. For most guys, that meant just lifting them off the floor and shrugging the shoulders a couple of times before dropping them back down. It was always impressive to watch someone lay on one of the creaking benches and press the "buck and a quarters" as they were known, up over their chest with ease.

At that time, gym etiquette meant that you allowed others to share equipment you were using because there was not much to begin with. Workout towels to wipe sweat off benches were not needed when you could easily wipe it away with your greasy blue jeans. No one dressed in gym clothes, just tank tops, blue jeans, and work boots. If you ever got thirsty you could find water around the back of the building in the form of a garden hose. This was my first experience with strength and conditioning, and I liked everything about it.

In 1991, I moved to Santa Cruz, California and found a job at a family-owned health club. It was a dream job for me. I was working in a gym and living by the beach in California. I got to meet hundreds of people and make great friends while helping them exercise. My days off were spent mountain biking in amazing terrain and surfing historic surf spots. Could it get any better? Within a few months the club began something new, a personal training program. It was something that the big city health clubs were doing and it was slowly trickling down to the suburbs. People would pay someone, on a regular basis, to guide them through their workouts. The concept sounded somewhat absurd. Who would pay to be told what they should already know how to do?

I jumped at the idea. Within a few months I became one of the first Certified Strength & Conditioning Specialists in Santa Cruz County. I discovered I loved studying movement. I could sit in on lectures and workshops and be engrossed the entire time. I became affiliated with the National Strength & Conditioning Association (NSCA). By the following year, the NSCA recognized that there was a future in personal training and created a certification specifically for personal trainers. I was one of the first to take the exam.

A year later, in 1995, I traveled to New Orleans for the NSCA National Conference. It proved to be a pivotal point in my young career. One of the presenters at the conference would later become my first mentor in helping me truly understand the importance of posture and the power of movement. Geoff Gluckman, of Dynamics of Physical Development Consultants, from San Diego, spoke of "Muscle Balance & Function Development." He spoke about the relevance of posture and maintaining a balance of tension between the muscles of the body. He explained how many of the exercises performed in gyms and health clubs were creating muscular imbalances and distorted posture. This could ultimately lead to pain symptoms such as tendinitis, bursitis, joint impingement, and bulging discs. Was this heresy or enlightenment? Could the bodybuilding style of resistance training we were giving our clients actually be doing harm? Did the joint problems that clients experienced, during and after the training session, relate to exercises they were given?

At that time, the standard operating procedure for joint or muscle pain was to avoid the exercise and choose a different one. For many clients, this led to an increasing number of exercises they did not perform. Were we just painting them into tighter corners? If barbell curls bothered somebody's elbow, the solution was to stretch the biceps and switch to dumbbells. Then, when the elbows began hurting with dumbbells, the answer was to stretch the biceps and lower the weight, or sit the person in a curling machine. It was the physical therapist's job to deal with pain. It did not matter that the client had not experienced pain before they began a personal training program.

I was forced to take a step back and look hard at what we were really doing to our clients. I began to realize that the programs were designed with the sole purpose of improving aesthetic qualities and not to improve function. This was reinforced by the clients themselves. Few people hired personal trainers to improve joint and muscle function. Almost everyone wanted a trainer to help them look better in the mirror. Therefore, program design took its cue from male bodybuilders and female fitness competitors. When it came to the clients who were competitive athletes, the programs did not change all that much. A few "sport-specific" exercises would be incorporated, but the majority of movements remained the same as the training program for women who wanted to get ready for bikini season.

After listening to Gluckman's entire lecture, it became obvious to me that I was achieving the antithesis of my goal. I was unknowingly creating programs that were hurting, rather than helping my clients. It became imperative that I change what I was doing and learn as much as I could from this man who pulled the veil away from my eyes. Geoff became my mentor for the next four years. He taught me how to perform posture assessments, to understand what a person's structure was doing in three dimensions, and which exercises would retrain the neuromuscular system so as to pull the body back into better alignment, strength, and joint function.

Up until that point, I had no idea that movement could remove pain. I knew that physical therapy helped people after surgeries and injuries, but this was different. Ice packs, soft tissue manipulation, and muscle stimulation machines were beyond a personal trainer's scope of practice. This new approach was simply giving someone exercises based on their posture, exercises that reduced postural distortions and improved the balance between muscles. No longer was I completely avoiding exercises which created pain in my clients. I had tools to use that often addressed the issue which caused the pain. I began to look for the underlying problem, rather than paint clients into more corners.

The training programs I designed changed dramatically. I moved away from the fancy resistance machines that were littered throughout the club. They seemed to be one of the leading culprits to pulling the body into distorted positions, in combination with the emergence of cell phones, laptops, and other technology. The health club machines also trained the body to move in unnatural ways, ways which a person would never find themselves doing during the normal course of their day. When would someone ever need to lie face down and forcefully drive both heels to their knees? When would someone ever need to sit in a chair and pull their straight legs together from a split position? When would someone ever need to pull a chest pad down into their thighs? I had never really questioned this before, but simply took it as the way we should exercise. These machines no longer made much sense. Yes, they trained muscles and would get people stronger doing the robotic movements, but if it was all they did, the price users would pay with joint or soft tissue pain seemed too great. I was tired of mindlessly following what the fitness culture was promoting at that time.

FUNCTIONAL TRAINING

As the new millennium approached, personal trainers shifted away from machine-based, isolated training, and the dawn of "functional training" began. The problem was, if you asked a dozen trainers what that meant, you would get a dozen different answers. The common bond in all of the answers was to train the body in ways in which the body functions. Functional training was meant to be a collection of exercises that trained individuals to perform the activities of daily life with more ease and fewer injuries. The primary actions of pushing, pulling, rotating, and moving up, down, and through space, were at the heart of functional movements. Ultimately, functional exercise focused most attention on the muscles surrounding the trunk and lower back and how they worked to allow force to transfer through the limbs. Traditional strength exercises were only selected if they resembled any type of daily movement. It was a good start to developing more full-body strength and conditioning programs, but it was still in an infancy stage. New "functional" equipment, such as stability balls and inflatable domes, poured into gyms and training studios. Old equipment such as kettlebells, medicine balls, and climbing ropes got dusted off and were now being used again. Medicine balls date back to the days of Hippocrates, kettlebells to 19th century Russia, and climbing ropes were in the gymnasiums of the mid-1800s. Tractor tires, sledgehammers, furniture dollies, and heavy ropes were converted into workout equipment, too. It seemed that hardware stores and yard sales were the perfect place to get the new exercise equipment.

In 1996, I left the health club to open my own training facility. My

new facility had some pieces of equipment that were still focused on aesthetics, because educating clients about posture and movement was not a quick process. Other equipment fell in the grey area of "functional training." With its growing popularity this "functional" approach became bastardized and soon would see trainers getting their clients to do ridiculous things like performing ultra-heavy barbell squats while standing on balance boards or inflatable stability balls. It almost seemed as if trainers were trying to outdo one another with novel routines. Fitness conventions began to resemble carnivals, trainers were performing single leg squats with a barbell on the shoulders while standing on a medicine ball, or jumping from one stability ball to another with dumbbells in hand. It appeared that many personal trainers had forgotten the purpose of "functional training" and replaced it with movements that nobody performed or needed. Fortunately, Facebook posts were not yet a reality because the insanity would have reached epidemic proportions. It reached its zenith for me when an issue of *Golf Digest* magazine pictured a professional golfer swinging his club while standing on a stability ball. Mainstream fitness was infected with this absurdity. I cannot say that I was immune. I do recall trying some stupid human tricks with a client or two. Luckily, it was a short-lived period and no clients were injured in the process.

A short while later, I was hired by a chiropractic clinic to provide realignment exercises to their patients. They saw that if the patients performed exercises immediately after chiropractic treatment, it resulted in decreased pain symptoms and it sped up rehabilitation. It also gave the patient tools which they could use on their own to be self-reliant and, in part, responsible for their own well-being. Training sessions at my facility were normally one hour long, but sessions at the chiropractic clinic were only thirty minutes, so I would typically see eight patients in a four-hour block. This forced me to condense the static posture assessment process, then create and implement a corrective strategy in a matter of minutes. It was kind of like speed dating, but matching up posture and exercise with a client's needs. The number of different physical issues ranged widely. People with all forms of joint issues and pain symptoms continually flowed through my exercise room. The knowledge and experience I gained was accelerated greatly. Inevitably, as my business continued to grow, I had to leave the chiropractic clinic, yet our referral network remains intact to this day.

MOVEMENT SCREENING

Up until this point in the fitness industry, there existed some standard assessments. Trainers would administer these assessments to gain an understanding of what the client needed and what elements should be in the client's training program. A maximal bench press or push-up test was used to establish upper body strength. A maximal leg press or squat test was used to determine lower body strength. A sit and reach test was used to test flexibility. A treadmill or bicycle test was normally used to establish aerobic capacity (the ability of the body to utilize oxygen as a fuel source). The tests were what every personal training certification process taught as the way to establish a baseline for fitness. The trouble with these tests was that they did not take into consideration the level of movement quality of the individual. All that was required was the ability to produce force any way possible. It was all about quantity, not quality. There was so much missing, but there was nothing available that trainers could use to gain a better sense of what each client really needed.

That is, until a couple of physical therapists and a chiropractor developed something called the Functional Movement Screen (FMS). It was the first system of its kind. Originally designed as a means of determining if high school athletes were ready for strength training, it was a system that would help identify muscular imbalances, movement restrictions, weaknesses, and compensations. It would help determine the amount of mobility and stability of the major joints in the body. When I combined this dynamic screening process with the static posture assessment, I gained a better understanding of which exercises would benefit clients the most.

The screens involved participants reaching behind their backs with one arm behind the head and the other behind the lower back. How close could the hands come to one another? Was it identical with opposite arms reaching? Another screen involved stepping over a rubber band that was positioned at knee level, while holding a plastic dowel across the shoulders and balancing on one leg. There was a screen that had the person hold the dowel directly overhead while attempting to squat very low. Another involved balancing on a 2x6 plank in a split stance with a dowel against the spine and lowering the back knee to the plank. This was a brilliant strategy to give personal trainers some gauge for measuring the ability of the client, instead of how much weight could they lift. However, it still seemed to be missing just one important piece: these were not movements people did on a daily basis or even in a sport! They were testing the ability of the particular movements and little else.

Almost every screen demanded awkward actions; most people were unfamiliar with them. Very few clients could successfully achieve the movements. The athletes we trained did well with the system but the general population failed horribly. Most could not perform the intense-style push-up or balance on the 2x6 board and lower to the floor. From a psychological or emotional perspective this was disastrous. The majority of people seek personal trainers because they feel bad, out of shape, and are not confident in their physical abilities. The last thing they needed was a process that proved they were what they felt: failures. As I sought more insight and understanding, I began to find other tools that worked better in my studio and with more clients.

Not long after, I was introduced to Gary Gray and the Gray Institute. Gary had been a successful physical therapist in Michigan for decades. He developed his own version of movement screens for personal trainers. It was quite simple and, in its simplicity, was brilliant. There were a total of six movements. Clients were asked to step forward and back, step to the left and right, and step in a rotating fashion left and right. The person's arms would also be reaching in the same or opposite direction as the stepping leg. All movements were achievable by everyone. Success was measured rather than failure. Trainers were instructed to find the movements which were the most successful and focus attention on them to help improve the areas which were less successful.

I dove into this approach with great enthusiasm. It helped me gain a better understanding of which exercises clients really needed to help improve their performance and reduce nagging pain. It also allowed me to narrow the gap which exists between the moment people are released from the care of a physical therapist and when they are ready to begin other exercise. The Gray Institute offered other courses and certifications that I greedily devoured as fast as I could. The other screening systems began to collect dust in the corner of the gym like toys my children had outgrown. One of the courses I enrolled in was titled "Chain Reaction."

It supplied better insight as to how each joint of the body moved and related to the other joints. Specifically, the course looked at gait (how the body acted and reacted when walking). It looked at what happens at the foot when it strikes the ground, and how that triggers a reaction at the ankle, knee, and hip.

Up until then, no matter which screening procedure I used, there was still one thing they were not assessing: *screening how the body traveled through space*. Every single one of the screening movements kept the body in one place. The limbs or torso might move but the body never left one central location. I felt this was a big piece of the puzzle that was not being considered. How does someone move from point A to point B? Would that not provide the trainer with valuable insight? People are not trees; they are not constantly anchored to the ground. They move. They walk. They run. Would it not make sense to gain a better understanding of how the primary means of locomotion was achieved? That saying of "walk before you can run," really rang true.

ENTER THE FOOT

At that time, the foot was not a hot topic in the fitness world. It seemed that it was considered just something that flapped along at the end of your leg. All the focus was on the hips, spine, and core. Even when I would perform the static posture assessment or the movement screens, I gave little consideration to the foot. How absurd is that? I feel like a fool when I think back to my lack of understanding. The one part of the body which contacts the planet thousands of times each day, and no one seemed all that interested in it. Never mind that the feet have more than 25 percent of the bones of the body and more than 60 joints, bones and joints that are meant to move in all directions with each step. It became clear to me: If something was not moving well at the feet, what kind of chain reaction would occur throughout the body?

Observing how someone walks was eye opening. It is a movement that almost every person on earth is familiar with, a movement that has evolved over millions of years. It is a pattern of movement which, similar to fingerprints, is unique to the individual, with no two people being identical. The average American takes 5,000 steps every day, or 1,825,000 a year! You don't perform any other full body action with the same regularity. Here, right under my nose all this time, was the ultimate screening method! I needed to learn more about the feet, human biomechanics (laws relating to movement or structure of people), and how I could use a person's gait pattern as an assessment tool.

Within a few months, my wish became a reality. I came upon an excerpt from a book titled, *What the Foot?: A Game-Changing Philosophy in Human Movement to Eliminate Pain and Maximize Human Potential.* One part of the excerpt stated that every bone in the body, during gait, should experience movement in three dimensions. The joints between the bones should also experience a freedom of movement through their appropriate range during some moment of the gait cycle (the movement the body experiences, while walking, when one heel strikes the ground until the same heel strikes the ground again). This meant that almost every joint motion should naturally occur when somcone walks, even if it is for a fraction of a second. So, if someone has a distortion in their posture, that means they are somehow stuck in some phase of the gait cycle. They do not get to experience how to properly enter and exit each phase. Getting the body to properly experience how to move in and out of each phase could help in reducing compensations and postural distortions, while improving joint function and overall performance.

I sent away for the book immediately. When it arrived in the mail,

I found a small insert inside the pages. It was a handwritten note from the author, Gary Ward, thanking me for the purchase. He also wrote that if I were interested in learning more, that I should attend one of his educational courses. He lived in London, but in just a few months would be offering his very first course in the United States. As luck would have it, the course was to take place just north of San Francisco, a 90-minute drive from my studio. What were the odds? Opportunity was not just knocking on the door, it was trying to bust it down. After reading the book, and having numerous epiphanies in the process, I signed up to take the course.

The course proved to be as promised. It was game-changing. Gary explained that he had mapped out how every single joint of the body moved in three-dimensional space through the entire gait cycle. He called it the *Flow Motion Model*®. Using his model, the students in the course were able to understand human movement at a level that was almost beyond comprehension. We could observe one joint of the body in its natural resting position and how it moved in space. By understanding the joint's ability (and inability) to move properly, we were able to theorize what all of the other joints in the body should be doing and observe which joints were not doing what they should. This was more or less like following clues to a mystery. We could take a step back and observe the entire body as it moved, or screen one joint in motion and get a better understanding of which exercises would be beneficial. Combining a static posture assessment with a dynamic gait analysis was even more of a complete picture.

Instead of this being another piece to my puzzle, it is more like the picture on the puzzle box. It is a map that allows me to know where to place all of the pieces. It opened the door to a world of greater understanding. Over the past six years of being under Gary's and his associate Chris Sritharan's, tutelage, I have been able to help hundreds of people who were plagued by chronic and acute pains and injuries. I have also been able to help athletes reach a higher level of performance. Many of these people had tried numerous Western and alternative approaches with little or no improvement. For many, all that was needed was to have their bodies experience long-forgotten movement. A physical awakening would take place and the body would respond in amazing ways, no matter how many years they had experienced pain.

As this journey and my studies with my mentors continue, another step along this educational path involves the world of motor neurology and how movement affects the brain and how the brain affects movement. Dr. Eric Cobb and his educational company known as Z-Health are leading the way in this "final frontier." For the past few years I have studied with this company and am thoroughly pleased with the tools I have been able to use under their guidance. We will touch upon some of the elements of motor neurology in this book, but I suggest you go directly to the source if you want more information. That is true for Anatomy in Motion and Gary Ward's work as well.

A BETTER WAY

The training programs we design in my studio, and which are described in this book, are dictated by the quality of a person's posture and gait motions, not on if they can step over a rubber band, balance on a plank, or how much they can bench press. We find out what someone has trouble doing and then give strength, mobility, or neurological exercises to access the movements. It does not matter if they are professional or Olympic-level athletes, or sedentary grandparents. The result is increased strength, increased mobility, improved muscular balance, improved posture, more energy, and a tremendous reduction or elimination of pain.

Most of the exercises in this book focus on *joint movement* rather than isolating a muscle or group of muscles. When a joint moves through space, all of the surrounding tissue has to react. Therefore, it is rather unfair to try and blame one specific muscle for all the body's problems. It has become popular in the fitness industry to place blame on just one muscle. Some instructors will tell clients that their problem is the gluteus medius (outer butt muscle) is weak and needs to be stronger. Others will blame the iliopsoas, or the abdominals, or the diaphragm, or a deep muscle along the spine called the multifidus. It appears that every few months a different muscle is to blame. Entire articles are written about one muscle and how imperative it is to make it stronger. It is very similar to fad diets. One month it's low carb, another it's high fat, the next it's high protein, and the next it's raw food. With more than 635 muscles in the body, do you really think one muscle is to blame for all your aches and pain? We are made up of 360 joints that are meant to move with relative ease with one another.

There needs to be a shift away from the old thought pattern of training muscles. It needs to be more about training *movement*. Muscles do not move in isolation. Movement is an integrative flow of energy between nerves, bones, tissues, and organs. When the body has the ability to move unrestricted, in all three dimensions, the muscles respond in kind. In order for the body to move in such a way, it needs to start from the right position: center! This is much like the hub of a bicycle wheel. When all of the spokes have an equal amount of tension, the hub is in its true spot, and the shape of the wheel is a perfect circle. True, perfect center is the position the body is in when all muscles maintain an equal balance of tension. It is when all joints are in their perfectly aligned resting posture.

It is when all internal organs and the neurological system are operating at their optimal level.

There are many elements which draw the body away from center. Injuries, scars, emotional trauma, chemical imbalances, disease, reduced activity levels, too much activity, and diminished organ function can all contribute to pulling the body away from center. The further the body travels away from true center, the weaker it becomes, the more diminished its potential. Therefore, as a trainer, no matter who I work with, the ultimate goal is always the same, return them closer to center. The closer we get to center, the stronger the body becomes, the better the body works, the less pain that is experienced, and the happier and healthier a person is. Workout programs need to be built around this philosophy. Guide a person back toward center. The ultimate goal is not to achieve a state of perfect balance, but simply to head in that direction.

TARGET THE PROBLEM, NOT THE SYMPTOM: A LESSON IN HISTORY

At one time my son and I were studying the Revolutionary War and the events leading up to it. We read about the Stamp Act, the Townshend Act, the Quartering Act, the Boston Massacre, and the Boston Tea Party. After studying these events he asked me why. Why did these things happen? I told him because the King of England wanted a debt repaid.

I explained that several years earlier the colonists were threatened from the north by the French and the native peoples, who attacked the colonists and tried to conquer their land. The King of England sent forces to the colonies to protect them. This cost a lot of money, which needed to be recouped. The king tried to get his money back by raising taxes on the colonists, but the colonists had other ideas and a revolution was born.

It is very important that we study history in order to understand where we find ourselves today. I relay this story because it is very similar to when a person develops pain in their body. There is always a reason for pain. It does not just appear on a whim. It is a reaction to some action or stimuli.

I had a man come see me who had been suffering from lower back pain for almost two years. He had tried several approaches (chiropractic, acupuncture, massage, and physical therapy) to addressing his pain and although some helped there was not one thing that was truly successful.

We began with making a timeline of all of his injuries, significant illnesses, accidents, etc., trying to get an idea of what occurred before the back pain and which might have led to where he now found himself. There was a basketball injury to his left leg 30 years earlier, back in his high school days. That was followed by surgery on his left knee to repair an injury he sustained while playing baseball not long after the first injury. There were some other episodes like a broken finger and impact to his right shoulder, but the high school injuries were what interested me the most.

When we captured his gait on video, we could see quite easily that he was not wanting to place much of his weight over his left leg. Even though his injury had occurred decades ago, his body was still moving like the injury had occurred yesterday. This was causing many of the muscles on his right side to undergo a lot more work to support him with every step he took. It also meant that his spine was having to adjust to living over his right leg and was never given a chance to experience what life was like over the left leg.

Could this gait pattern have been created 30 years ago and never gone away? The answer is yes. Remember, it took 13 years after the French & Indian War ended for Thomas Jefferson to write the Declaration of Independence. It might take 13 years for pain to develop from an early injury. Unless proper movement patterns get reestablished, the strategy the subconscious mind develops to stay away from pain and future injury will continue. We began training his body to load weight onto his left side and developed a strength program based on his gait pattern and what was missing. The pain diminished during the first session. Before long the pain was gone. It was by figuring out how his body moved that we were able to create a specific conditioning program for him. He had performed countless workouts in the past before coming to see me, but they were all generic with no specificity for his imbalances and gait pattern.

CHAPTER 1
WHAT IS MISSING?

THE EFFECTS OF LIVING IN THE MODERN WORLD

Living in a technologically advanced society comes at a price. With the demand for purposeful, physical activity at an all-time low, there are more laborsaving and time-saving devices on the market than ever. At one time people had to grow and hunt their food, yet in today's world, they can use their thumbs and order dinner on their smart phone and have the food delivered while they sit and watch television. If standing in line at the coffee shop for the caramel capufrachiato is too tiring, they can use their smart phone at the table and place the order. For some, even having to hold the smart phone is too much and they just speak into their watch. They can order anything with a simple turn of the wrist and a few words. The human body is not being used the way it evolved to be used. Now, it is evolving to meet the needs of this new existence. We see it all around us. There are more people who are overweight or obese than those who are not. Injuries are occurring at younger ages, as are health issues related to lifestyle choices. Bodies are breaking down and something needs to be done about it.

PITFALLS OF CONVENTIONAL STRENGTH TRAINING PROGRAMS

Currently, the majority of strength exercises found in a gym are well documented and have the potential to be positive: increased bone density, elevated metabolism, enhanced muscular strength and endurance, greater production of the human growth hormone, and improved self-confidence. However, the approach to strength training and how a person utilizes the exercises can have several shortcomings over time. When we move (walk, run, play sports) we do so by swinging our limbs in opposite directions. So why are the majority of strength exercises performed bilaterally, such as squats, bench presses, barbell curls, or pull-ups? Almost every circuit machine in a gym encourages bilateral action, too. The leg press, leg extension, leg curl, pec deck, inner/outer thigh, and deltoid fly machines all encourage both arms or legs to move in unison in the same direction. Even dumbbells, which can be used with freedom of limb action, often are used together in the same direction at the same time.

The goal for many exercise enthusiasts is to create symmetry: a balance of tension, shape, and size to the muscles. At first thought, it makes sense to create a training program comprised mainly of bilateral actions. Bilateral movements ask an equal amount of work, but the way each side, or limb, generates the force required may be quite different. Bilateral movements expect the person performing the movements to be perfectly balanced, centered, and aligned, just like the image in an anatomy book. Yet, it would be extremely rare to find a person who is truly balanced, orbiting around true center, and whose structure is ideally aligned. Injuries, surgeries, and a whole range of other elements pull the body away from this perfect space. So, even though the body overall will grow stronger, the training programs unknowingly reinforce muscular imbalances. Therefore, the way in which each movement is executed will be compromised and the degree of compensation will be dependent upon how the whole body moves with all of its imbalances and restrictions. The resulting effect will be a body that is structurally compromised, that trains under greater and greater loads. It is similar to the family game where rows of rectangular wooden pieces are stacked in opposing directions to make a small tower. As one piece is removed and placed on top, the tower's center of mass rises and the structure becomes more compromised. All it takes is one piece to be dropped in just the wrong place, and the tower comes crumbling down.

When the body is in motion it does not move by recruiting both legs forward at the same time (unless you live in a rowboat). When the body moves, the arms swing in opposing directions. The legs swing in concert with the arms. The torso rotates due to the swinging limbs. The spine will flex, extend, side bend, and rotate. Bilateral exercises prohibit most of these actions. Focusing strength training programs mainly on bilateral movement neglects how the body moves the majority of the time. A program heavily biased to bilateral action is like placing a gag order on the spine; it sends confusing signals to the brain when the body needs to travel through space. Humans spend most of their waking hours moving by shifting their weight from one side to the other. Very little time is spent balanced evenly over both feet. Bilateral strength training negates rotation and lateral action, and often requires the spine to be as static as possible.

This is great when you are in the process of lifting heavy objects up and down, but what about when you are playing tennis, dodging defenders on a football field, or reaching in the trunk of the car to grab groceries? Granted, there are many times when we find the need to push something with both arms. We get up and down from the chair with both legs at the same time. However, we move so much more by having our limbs move in opposition, if we don't make the majority of the strength routine reflect that, we are missing the target.

Then there are strength imbalances. Typically, one arm is stronger than the other and one leg is stronger than the other. The muscles in the front of the waist often will relax and get longer while the muscles of the lower back shorten to take on a greater load of work to support excess weight in front. These common, simple strength imbalances will continue to exist, even though one may begin to build strength. The body will be able to produce a greater degree of force, but with the same diminished structural integrity. Traditional exercises are not necessarily going to correct the imbalances, but they will have a greater chance of further pulling a person's structure out of alignment. This also does not take into consideration any existing conditions, previous injuries, or surgeries which might further affect the body's ability to move perfectly. This could lead to problems.

Most traditional exercises can be performed in a very narrow space. Pushdowns, pulldowns, curls, deadlifts, squats, step-ups, push-ups, dips, shoulder presses, and lunges can all be done inside a tall door frame. Most of these motions move in primarily one dimension and do not require much from the other two dimensions (lateral or rotational motion). This is very biased and is extremely limiting. As humans, we are meant to move in three-dimensional space and in multiple directions. Watch a person put away their groceries or load the washing machine or take a load out of the dryer. Think of how a basketball player or tennis player moves on the court. None of these actions are strictly linear. Often, the moves are a combination of side bending, reaching, and rotating. Yet, even many of these athletes spend most of the time in the gym stuck in the forward and backward dimension of movement known as the sagittal plane. What might happen if they reduced the number of bilateral, linear movements and trained multidimensionally? Would their bodies be more fluid and better prepared to handle the infinite combinations of movements available? Might we see a drop in non-contact sports injuries, and aches and pains of everyday living?

The primary purpose in most training programs is to build strength by imposing a demand to produce force in the body any way possible, until it begins to fatigue. This is known as the SAID Principle. SAID stands for **S**pecific **A**daptations to **I**mposed **D**emands. This means that the body will be forced to change based on what it encounters. If you are always training the bench press, you will get very good at pressing a heavy bar off your chest. How many times in real life, outside of your training program, will that be necessary? Perhaps if you are a wrestler and need to press your opponent off when he or she is on top of you and you are lying on your back. But then again, that means you are pinned and the match is over. This is not to paint the picture that the bench press is a bad exercise or to disparage any and all of the other bilateral movements. It just serves to point out that there might be other movements a person might want to encourage and develop, movements that are more related to their sport or their activities of daily life.

MUSCULAR IMBALANCES

Imagine two people digging a hole. One person is larger and stronger and has been a professional ditch digger for many years. Both people keep the same pace with their shovels, but the stronger individual is more efficient, more practiced, and because he is good natured, loads his shovel with more earth to help the other person complete the hole. Both might appear to be performing the same work, but that is not the case.

Few people are truly ambidextrous, so one arm is usually used and developed more than its counterpart. Two different neurological patterns of motion develop, like the difference between writing your name with each hand. That means the muscles of the arms will develop a bit differently. Most people have a preferred leg with which they kick a ball. This develops two different roles for the leg: one is the stabilizer, and the other creates brute force to send the ball flying. This also helps encourage subtle rotations, and shifts the body's center of mass away from a true balanced point.

What is the outcome, over the course of time, of performing squats, deadlifts, or some other bilateral exercise with such a situation? This also equates to performing a unilateral exercise on one side of the body and then the other. The way in which the body would coordinate the muscle action will be quite different. You see it all the time but might not realize it. Have you ever noticed someone performing a barbell squat, and as the hips descend, they begin to shift the hips over one foot more than the other? How many people do you see perform the bench press and one elbow flares out wider than the other, or one hand is closer to the center of the bar than the other? Perhaps there is a subtle tilt of the bar toward the stronger side. The more this is repeated the more the differences between the sides are reinforced, not corrected. This uneven muscular development is the cause of many joint issues.

What this means, contrary to popular opinion, is that you may not need to perform the same exercise or amount of work on each side of the body with every lift. One side of the body, or one motion, may need additional time to improve control, efficiency, and coordination. You may need to do more work on one side than the other to bring the weaker side up to the same strength level as the dominant side. It is essential that a better balance of strength and mobility be developed first, before encouraging balanced, bilateral or alternating motions, on both sides.

HIGHLY REPETITIVE ACTIONS AND WEAR PATTERNS

Traditional strength exercises are meant to be performed with a high degree of repetition; if not during the workout itself, then over weeks and weeks of workouts. What happens to carpeting in the house of a family of five over the course of years? It begins to develop wear patterns. The carpet fibers are pushed down every time a foot comes crashing down. The more this happens, the more the fibers wear down and tear. Eventually, a wear pattern emerges and it becomes obvious which rooms have the most traffic and where nobody ever steps. The same can occur in the body, especially in the joints, muscles, and soft tissues. Most people select the exercises they most enjoy, and they perform these exercises more often than others. They become very good and strong with these specific movements; this makes them want to do the same exercises even more. After some time (months, years, decades?) the wear pattern becomes apparent. Inflammation, joint restriction, and discomfort begin to develop somewhere. The overstimulated muscles generate a greater-than-average force and begin to pull the person off center. Their posture becomes compromised. The body must adapt to the change. Discomfort turns into pain and now the once-favorite exercise needs to be modified. This is typically when the aging process is blamed. Really? What if you regularly changed strength exercises and explored new movements? Rather than relying on the same strengths over time, what if you explored weaker movements which could be developed to become just as strong? That is, explore the areas of carpet less traveled. Make all the weak links better in the chain! Cover the whole carpet.

Strength training can bring the body back to a more centered, posturally aligned, highly functional state. If used properly, it can eliminate pain, instead of creating it. Strength training can improve so many things, even organ function; it just needs to be used with better precision and understanding.

WHAT IS MISSING?

By knowing what strength training can provide, along with its shortcomings, we can gain a better understanding of what is missing. It is time to fill in the gaps and design programs that address missing elements. So, what are these elements?

INTEGRATE MORE THAN ISOLATE

The primary goal of modern competitive bodybuilding is to display and improve the aesthetic quality and size of muscles. This goal is primarily achieved by isolating the largest muscles to develop more definition and hypertrophy (the increase of muscle fiber size). During the onset of the fitness revolution, when it came time to develop exercise machines, the engineers recruited the help of the guys who were already in the gyms—the bodybuilders. Health clubs and gyms began to take on a much different look. Instead of racks of dumbbells and barbells along the walls, and universal, multipurpose cable systems in the center of the room, the facilities were filled with rows and rows of fancy, upholstered equipment. Little placards attached to each machine depicted what big muscle the machine would target, and gave instructions on how to use the machine. This reduced the need for and cost of having instructors in the exercise areas, which pleased the gym owners even more.

Most machines required participants to lie face up or face down, or be seated, while they pushed or pulled in order to produce force in the

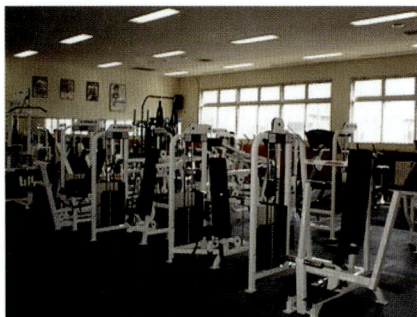

target area. Wasn't the problem that Americans were already lying down or sitting too much as it was? Wasn't the lack of purposeful physical movement the reason why gyms and health clubs were exploding on the scene? The breakdown in logic continued on for decades. This is not to say that machines are all bad. They serve a valid purpose in getting people to move more, but too much of anything is not ideal.

The shortcomings of the machines, and there are many, eventually came to light in the late 1990s. It became obvious that the machine-based movements did not strengthen the way people actually moved in daily life. Rarely would a person need to sit in a chair and forcefully drive their

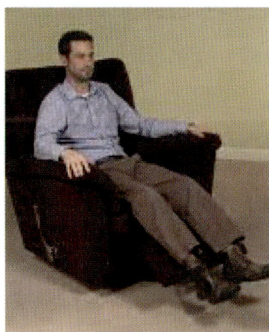

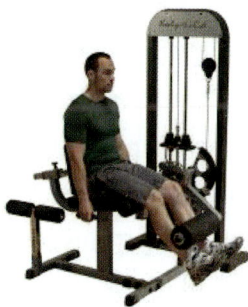

heels underneath the seat like that of the leg curl machine, unless they had a stubborn recliner. There would be few times a person might need to lean back in a chair and force their straight legs open and closed as they do on the inner and outer thigh machines. Unless you are a parent of a toddler, chances are you do not need to sit in a chair and bounce weights up on the shins and ankles as you do on the leg extension machine.

Aside from the unnatural movements the machines reinforced, they also created a greater potential for muscular imbalances, which happens when some muscles contract more than their counterpart. As explained previously, when muscular imbalances increase, joint position is compromised, compensation increases, and the body alters the way it moves. Over time, the imbalances lead to distorted posture, joint pain, and soft tissue inflammation. It became quite common for gym goers to experience shoulder impingement, tennis elbow, knee pain, and an assortment of other orthopedic maladies.

Most of the machines focused on producing force in one region and keeping it from flowing through the rest of the body. Also removed from training was the need for coordination and balance. Very little coordination and balance are required to operate a machine. Trainers coached clients to maintain a rigid stance, or seated position, with little extraneous motion; just isolate that area…feel the burn! The more this is reinforced, the less the body is able to transfer force from head to toe. The smaller stabilizing muscles that help transfer force from the arms, to the trunk, and down the legs, were neglected. The big muscles gain size and the smaller muscles are overwhelmed and unfamiliar with how to handle the increased strength level of the larger muscles. In essence, they get beat up like a little kid against the school-yard bully. To address these aches and pains, sports medicine doctors began setting up shop near every gym. A steady stream of patients came in complaining of rotator cuff issues, low back pain, groin pulls, golfer's elbow, and a host of other injuries. Neoprene sleeves appeared on elbows, knees, and ankles, and a new fashion statement became en vogue. The way America was training was more for display and not for functional everyday life.

To this day, the majority of health clubs (and physical therapy clinics) still fill their facilities with isolating strength machines and have their staff place club members in every single one. It is so much easier to place members on machines than it is to teach them how to properly move their bodies or lift the free weights. Therefore, a large number of gym members almost exclusively work out on just the machines. The next thing you know is they get injured, and their attendance craters. The gym owner does not necessarily mind because the member is still paying their monthly dues. In fact, that makes the gym less busy and allows new members to fill the gap. The members drop but the profits soar.

Rather than develop a program that focuses on specific muscles, it is better to *focus on specific movements*. We do not move by isolating a muscle, so to only train in that way does not help improve overall movement. Sitting in a leg extension machine and building stronger quadriceps muscles will not help someone reach in the dryer with a heavy load of wet clothes. By focusing on complex movements, the muscles and the rest of the body learn the proper timing patterns to perform the movements successfully. This is a synergistic way of learning and developing.

SELECT EXERCISES BASED ON THE INDIVIDUAL'S STRUCTURE AND GAIT PATTERN

If we seek to improve performance, for any activity, would it not make sense to begin at one of the most basic, common actions known to man? If proper joint relationships are not occurring in gait, how can one expect proper movement to occur when running around a track, or playing basketball, swinging a golf club, or taking groceries out of the trunk of the car? By training proper joint mechanics, and reeducating and strengthening the muscles that react to them, a person will move with more efficiency, power, dynamic stability, and coordination. The exercise that you select will either encourage better movement or just the opposite.

Undertaking an exercise program without knowing how you move and what is missing in your movement is just rolling the dice and hoping for the best. If done poorly, the chance of creating greater imbalances, compensations, and injuries are much higher. The *Return to Center* method is based on the phases of the gait cycle and the corresponding joint coupling relationships. It is by reinforcing the biomechanics, and applying resistance or assistance when needed, that the body is able to get stronger in a way that improves overall performance with less chance of injury. Selecting exercises based on an individual's posture, muscular imbalances, quality of joint motion, and how they walk is much more beneficial and effective at restoring the body back to a more structurally aligned position and higher level of functionality and performance. After all, the human structure has evolved to walk over the past two million years. It is the fundamental, biomechanical means of getting from one place to another.

BE OKAY WITH WORKING JUST ONE SIDE

We must break away from the "Balance Myth" that suggests you always have to do the same exercise to both sides of the body. A body that is asymmetrical will not necessarily become symmetrical just because the same movement is performed on both sides. Even if both sides develop more strength, the stronger side will still remain the stronger side. It may be more effective to focus on one side to bring the body back to center.

HAVE A PROGRAM THAT CHANGES
WITH THE BODY

Because the brain, the body, and its posture are constantly adapting to the surrounding world, it does not seem logical that the same routine, over an extended period of time, would be as effective as would a continually changing routine that addresses the adaptations. Malleable programs that continually change based on the state of the body and how it organizes movement against gravity enables greater adaptations in the body and brain.

ASSESS AND REASSESS

A program that regularly encourages assessing and reassessing a person's quality of motion, optimal amount of resistance, and volume of work is needed. Assessing each movement tells us if we are on the right track, or if the movement is not what we need at that time. If we are not assessing then we are simply guessing. Removing the guesswork improves the quality of training.

LISTEN TO THE BRAIN

The brain is the overall governing system of the body. It constantly receives, interprets, and reacts to everything the body encounters, including exercise. One of its abilities is to control and regulate force output of muscles based on interpretation of stimuli. The brain will determine if the level of intensity (resistance) and volume (amount of work) is appropriate or if it considers it more of a threat. If the brain senses a threat, it will dampen the force output and impose greater limits on movement. A threat can manifest in several ways. Injured tissue or bone, restricted joints, improper posture, and compensatory movements can all be interpreted as threats in the brain. Efficient neurology is essential in force production. It is by relying on this neural feedback, known as the *Autonomic Nervous System*, that we can determine intensity and volume of any exercise. Simple range of motion assessments can be used as barometers to guide further progress.

BALANCE, MOBILITY, AND STRENGTH

There are three ways in which to build muscular strength: increase muscle size (hypertrophy), improve joint mechanics, and increase neural activation. A strength training program focused on gaining strength by overloading muscle with resistance and gaining hypertrophy often sacrifices joint mobility and neural activation. It takes weeks for muscles to build size, and if someone were to gain more than five pounds of muscle mass, this would be above average. More often, strength training gets the existing muscles to work harder and become more efficient. The nervous system is the overall governing system. If the joints move properly, there is less of a likelihood of a threat response and the muscles are able to produce much more force. Thus, creating a balance with the three elements of better joint mechanics, increased muscle size, and neural activation brings about greater strength levels and performance.

EXERCISES THAT IMPROVE THE NEURAL MAP

The connection between the musculoskeletal system and the nervous system needs to constantly be fine-tuned. Feeding multidimensional movement to the entire body and not just a few robotic, repetitive actions helps supply the brain with a better connection to the entire body. This is known as the neural map. Exploring all three dimensions of movement throughout the entire body awakens those nerve cells that lie in a somewhat dormant state. Dusting off the brain's neural map of where the body is in space will improve the ability to move, coordinate, and balance. This will in turn allow the brain to increase muscular force and utilize more of the existing strength within the body.

WHAT TO DO ABOUT IT

There is hope. Muscles can achieve a better level of balance. Joints can function more effectively and inflammation can be reduced. You just need to be given the tools to make this happen. By encouraging the neuromuscular and skeletal systems to experience proper, efficient movements, posture can be better aligned. This does not mean that everyone should think about standing tall, sitting upright, and not slouching. It's a nice idea but it is impossible to maintain consciously for even a moment. There are 206 bones, 360 joints, and more than 635 muscles in the body. No one can consciously control all of that and still be able to take a single step. Fortunately, our subconscious mind takes care of this for us. It is more a matter of sending the proper signals to the subconscious mind so it can better regulate efficient control.

This also does not mean you should head to the gym and begin bench pressing and squatting. It does not mean that everyone should take a yoga class or join a masters swim class. Exercise for the sake of exercise is great, but not every exercise is beneficial for everybody. One person might have weakness in one area while another person has it somewhere else. Performing push-ups, for example, may prove to be good for one person and detrimental for another. That is why following a generic workout routine found in a health and fitness magazine or online may be hazardous to your health.

TARGET THE PROBLEM, NOT THE SYMPTOM: FROZEN SHOULDER

A hairstylist at a nearby salon came to see me because of chronic pain in her right shoulder. It was just a little nagging sort of thing for the past few years, but lately the pain had grown to be too much. She couldn't lift her arm higher than a few inches. Reaching back behind her, such as reaching for a purse on the back seat of her car, was something she had not been able to do in over a year. She had to go home early from work the day before because of the pain. This was serious, because it involved her livelihood; if she could not lift her arms to cut hair she was out of income and out of business. She had tried a few things, like muscle rubs and massage, but those only gave her temporary relief.

She shared her history of injuries with me. She had broken her right wrist in high school; it had been placed in a cast. She also fractured the big toe of her left foot ten years earlier; that had required surgery and metal pins. She explained that her left sacroiliac joint felt jammed and that she had gone through a hysterectomy a couple of years ago.

One or more of these previous experiences could very well have contributed to her shoulder pain. If her broken wrist did not have its proper range of motion restored, it may have asked other areas to work harder, and over time, could have made another area irritated or inflamed. The hysterectomy left a small scar and even though it was fully healed without any complications, it could still have affected her structure. Her body could have been imperceptibly pulled toward the scar as a way of protecting itself, and that could have placed her shoulder in a compromised position for repetitive motions of cutting hair. As it turned out, the trouble seemed to have originated from the broken toe of her left foot.

As we directed our attention to her foot, she remembered something important (as it often occurs when "discarded" areas of the body begin to move again). She explained that after her foot surgery, she had suffered a fall and dislodged the metal pins through the sole of her foot. The pins pierced the skin through the bottom of her foot! That was pretty significant information. As a result, the pins were fully removed (in general, the fewer metal pins in the body the better), but she was, unknowingly, not willing to fully place weight on that forefoot. Chances are nobody would want to step on a place where, the last time you did, metal pins came shooting out.

We then noticed that she couldn't lift her big toe off the floor. That may not seem to be a big deal, but if she could not lift her big toe then she would be unable to properly supinate (create an arch in the foot). Without proper supination, she would struggle to create the proper chain reaction of joint and muscle movements above. She would struggle to extend her left knee or rotate her pelvis left, which would unlock the "jammed" sacroiliac joint. If the hips had difficulty rotating left, then her ribs would have trouble rotating right. When the ribs rotate right it allows the shoulder to retract, depress, rotate, and open up.

We found that by placing a small foam wedge under her big toe on the left foot, which gave her forefoot something to place weight upon, her right arm range of motion improved significantly! She was pretty blown away. This showed that the connection between the left foot and right shoulder function was worth exploring. We went through two exercises that explored integrative, full-body gait-specific motion. When she relearned how to transfer weight onto her left foot, she was able to experience her ribs rotating opposite her hips and that's when things really began to happen. What is interesting is that we did not focus on her shoulder and left it relaxed through the exercises.

After these movements she walked around. Then, we rechecked her shoulder pain and her arm's range of motion. Her jaw dropped and eyes went wide as she went through a full range of motion with no pain!!! For the first time in a year, she could reach back behind her without pain. This all took a grand total of 20 minutes. The problem was not her shoulder, but how her whole body was off center and had organized compensatory movement. We then selected several strength training movements to build up the weaker areas and a few mobility drills to open the restricted regions. Since then, she has not had the debilitating shoulder pain return. By bringing her structure back to center, pain disappeared and function was restored.

CHAPTER 2
WHAT IS CENTER, WHY IS IT IMPORTANT?

CENTER AND POSTURAL ALIGNMENT

When the body is in a state of perfect, balanced posture, everything is in its most ideal, central place. This system of balance has developed over the past two million years, ever since humans rose up on two feet.

The three-dimensional structural design of the human frame is much like a skyscraper. When the body stands in a resting posture each major load-bearing joint is designed to maintain right angles from all directions. Muscles and other connective tissues have just the right balance of tension (not too short or too long) to keep the bones in a structurally sound position. The bones maintain the ideal spacing from each other (not too close and not too far) so joint functions are at their highest potential for optimal movement. The internal organs are situated in just the right spot without any crimping, impingement, or excess tension. The nervous system receives and transmits the proper amount of stimuli to the entire body.

Think of this state of balance as the "Goldilocks Spot." Not too far left or right. Not too far forward or back. Not turning more to the left than to the right or vice versa. This is an almost mythological place that is nearly impossible to obtain in today's technologically advanced culture. Nonetheless, the closer the body gets to a balanced state, the better its overall performance. That is, therefore, the ultimate goal: to come as close as possible to a balanced state of being.

The trouble is, most people feel they have good posture, but what they may not be aware of is at some point their posture subtly shifted off center, and where they find themselves currently feels normal, but really is not.

Not long ago, some friends came into town, and when they saw my kids they couldn't get over how much they had grown. We made the typical nodding response of agreement, but then it got me thinking. Why don't we make the same exclamatory remark every time we see our kids? I mean they are constantly growing. Obviously, it is because the growth is gradual, and it is only over the course of some time that it is noticeable to the eye. The same can be said of how our body structure changes and adapts to our experiences and surroundings. We do not typically find ourselves with off-centered posture overnight. It is a subtle, insidious adaptation. The difference between kids growing up and a change in posture is that you can do something about your posture.

Movement is the key to improving posture; lack of movement means your posture will degrade even more. Improving your posture could very well depend on the type of movement you choose. Often, people will choose movements that reinforce the distortions rather than correct them. For instance, someone who sits at a desk all day will most likely have rounded shoulders, bent elbows, flexed hips, and a forward head position (in essence the more they sit, the more their posture adapts to sitting). Over time this posture normalizes.

This person may go to the gym, but the exercises they select may encourage more rounding of the shoulders, bent elbows, etc. They spend the majority of their workout doing bench presses, bicep curls, leg presses, and crunches. All of these movements reinforce excessive compression in the areas that are already neurologically shortened during their work day. Little do most people know that their workout is exacerbating the pains that come from distorted posture. It is a slow and insidious process that takes time to witness; the unchanging, repetitive nature of the exercises are rarely ever seen as the culprit. Therefore, the exercises people perform at the gym should be chosen based on what their structure is doing and the areas that do not receive as much stimuli.

It is these areas, nicknamed "dark zones," which need more attention. The "dark zones" are areas of the body that do not get a lot of stimuli due to distorted postures and compensatory motions. They remain under-stimulated, weak, and unused, or when they are used, they are used improperly. Ultimately, the goal of a workout is to achieve a greater balance of muscular tension, improved posture, and overall function. Finding the points of structural weakness and regions of excessive stress and strain are important pieces of information when designing a complete workout.

So how do you know which exercises will benefit *you*, and which will make your situation worse? First, you need an assessment of how you support your frame and how you move it. By "interviewing" the body, and getting a better understanding of these things, you can then select the movements best suited for you at this time. Remember, the body is always adapting to its environment. This means that the exercises you performed last month or last year may not be the best ones to do right now. A lot has happened in the past year. A lot has happened since last week! Do not get stuck, as many do, in performing the same routine over and over. Look what happens to carpet in the hallway. Walking the same pattern over and over eventually wears down the fabric and things begin to tear until you have to get new carpeting.

You want to continually adjust your training program to how your body responds to the world around you. Also, remember that you may get very adept at doing specific motions, but that means there are many more motions you are not practicing. You are only as strong as your weakest link.

CENTER OF MASS

The center of mass is the relative position of the average mass of all parts of a system. In the case of the human body, the center of mass is the point where the mean weight of all parts of the body meet; halfway between top and bottom, left and right, front and back. When a body is standing, in its most structurally balanced point, the center of mass is located approximately 10 centimeters below the navel, just above the hips. If you dropped a line straight

Sagittal
Frontal
Transverse
Planes of Movement

Human body with three planes of motion and indicating center of mass down, the point would be evenly between both feet. Generally speaking, the center of mass is near the fourth lumbar vertebrae. This point will vary slightly from one person to another because of shape, size, and gender. But what happens when joints shift and some muscles are forced to lengthen more than others and alter the position of the center of mass? The center migrates away from the fourth lumbar vertebrae in the direction of the shifting mass. No matter which joint is experiencing displacement, every other joint in the body must now alter its position and the muscles must adapt by lengthening or shortening to accommodate the changes. When one thing changes, everything changes.

This is similar to the hub of a bicycle wheel. All of the wheel's spokes come together and meet at the hub. The hub's position is dictated by the tension in the spokes. If all of the spokes have an equal amount of tension, then the hub is in its ideal central position, the wheel is a perfect circle, and the ride is as smooth as can be. But what if there is a spoke or two that have more tension than the others? That greater amount of tension will affect all of the other spokes, as they will be pulled more than normal. This, in turn, will shift the hub's position out of its ideal place. The further it travels from the ideal central spot, the more warped and weaker the wheel becomes. Even if it is just a hint of change the entire wheel shape will change. This will make the bike ride a bit bumpier and increase the wear on the entire bicycle. If the rider would "true up" the spokes and return them all to an equal balance of tension, the wheel's perfect circle would be restored and the ride would be smooth once more.

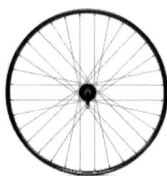

The muscles and soft tissue that surround the hips and pelvis are very similar. If there is a balance of tension top to bottom, left to right, and side to side, the position of the pelvis and all surrounding joints will be in their respective centers. This should occur with the muscles that surround every joint of the body. There would be the least amount of torque, and everything would maintain a neutral resting posture. The way in which a person moves would require the least amount of effort, stress, and wear-and-tear. The body's hub (center of mass and origin of motion) should ideally sit an inch or two in front of the disc between the fourth and fifth lumbar vertebrae. When the muscles are not balanced (due to adapting to sedentary environments, overuse, previous injuries, or surgeries and scarring) the center is pulled askew. If the center of mass is meant to hover near the fourth lumbar vertebra, how much pressure will be applied to that area if the center were to shift? Is it any wonder that up to 80 percent of the population will experience back pain at some time in their lives? How many people do you know with lower back pain? For many, it is simply because their center of mass has shifted, for whatever reason, resulting in a compromised, weaker, and more vulnerable structure. Consider that the pain symptom may not necessarily be located at the lower back. It could very well manifest anywhere in the body. The conventional approach to pain is to treat the pain site. But what if the pain is being caused by something that is out of place somewhere else? This is incredibly common and is why people continue to have joint pain even after taking anti-inflammatories, pain killers, and seeing medical professionals who hold on to the symptom-based approach, rather than looking for the true culprit.

> **Here are some of the potential issues and injuries that may appear when adaptations to posture become distorted and joint motion is compromised:**
>
> - Bursitis and Tendinitis (wrists, elbows, shoulders, etc.)
> - Plantar Fasciitis
> - Knee Pain
> - ACL Tear
> - Sciatica
> - Piriformis Syndrome
> - Scoliosis
> - Low Back Pain
> - Herniated or Ruptured Disc
> - Rotator Cuff Injuries
> - Shoulder Pain
> - Neck Pain
> - Migraines/Headaches
> - Tennis and/or Golfer's Elbow
> - Carpal Tunnel Syndrome
> - Dizziness
> - Bunions
> - Hammertoes

Whether it is the way in which the joints organize patterns of movement or muscles acting in a compensatory fashion is debatable, and ultimately, doesn't matter. The goal for strength, function, and pain elimination is to direct the body back to a more central point. The closer the body gets to "truing up" its spokes, the more optimally it will function, the greater the performance potential, and the more likely existing pain will disappear.

SHIFTING OFF CENTER

As I mentioned earlier, there are many elements that have the potential to drive us away from center. Injuries, surgeries, repetitive motions, illnesses, infections, neurological deficits, emotional trauma, chemical imbalances, and birthing issues are just some ways the body will be pulled away from center. Whenever the body suffers an injury, it subconsciously responds and adapts in such a way that it finds the

> No matter where the body determines where center is, it will constantly attempt to maintain an orbit around that center.

best way to survive and get around the pain (e.g., limping, leaning, twisting, etc.). With most injuries, eventually the pain subsides, but that does not mean that the body returns to where it was before the injury. In most cases, the body maintains a shadow of the compensatory movements it developed and reinforced when it was injured. There is no magic reset button that gets pressed just because the pain disappears. The body does not return to a balanced state.

This means that for every injury, surgery, illness, repetitive motion, etc. the body experiences, a new layer of compensation is created. The most recent episodes are layered on top of earlier experiences. This is why old injuries, which many people disregard because they were so long ago,

are very important to take into consideration. Many times, in order to bring the body back to center, it is the oldest injuries and experiences that need to be addressed rather than the more recent ones. Unless proper motion is reintroduced to the body, future injuries and pain have a much greater chance of occurring.

A person with a distorted posture.

FIVE RULES OF ANATOMY IN MOTION®

There are natural laws that govern our bodies. Simply put, it is all about gravity, mass, momentum, and ground reaction force. How does the human body act in the presence of gravity? How does it deal with moving its mass and controlling the momentum it creates? To better understand these concepts, we can look at the five rules of Anatomy in Motion® as presented by its founder, Gary Ward.

The five rules are:
• Muscles lengthen before they contract.

- Joints act, muscles react.
- Everything revolves around center.
- Perceived center dictates posture, performance, and potential.
- The brain is hardwired for perfection.

RULE #1. MUSCLES LENGTHEN BEFORE THEY CONTRACT

When the body is in motion, muscles act very much like rubber bands. In order to generate force and propulsion, they lengthen before they shorten. When someone jumps off the ground, they must first lower the body and lengthen the muscles, before shortening the muscles and driving off the ground.

This is known as the stretch-shortening reflex. Nerve cells called proprioceptors or mechanoreceptors tell the nervous system that the muscle tissue is lengthening. The nervous system tells the muscles to contract as they lengthen, to control the rate of length. This is, in part, a protective response to prevent damage to muscle tissue, connective tissues, and joints, as well as a way of managing mass and momentum.

This is followed by another message to shorten the muscles, to change the body's direction of motion, and propel it somewhere else. This occurs every time we take a step when walking and running.

We could view how a muscle contracts on a spectrum. On the left side of the spectrum is the shortening phase of the muscle known as a concentric contraction. On the right side is the lengthening phase of the muscle known as the eccentric contraction. Directly in the center of the spectrum is

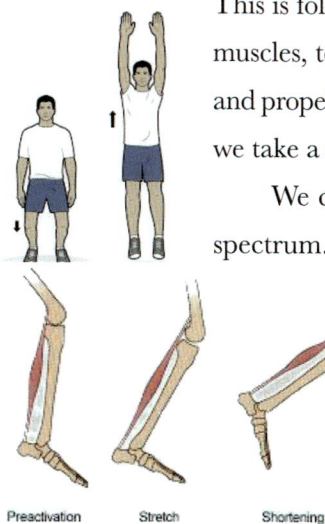

Preactivation   Stretch   Shortening

neutral, neither lengthening or shortening. In order for the body to move, it must travel to the right on the spectrum before traveling left. Most traditional strength exercises, as well as Pilates-based exercises, begin at neutral and travel into the concentric end of the spectrum, placing the emphasis of the muscle contraction on the shortening phase, spending the majority of time keeping the bones close together, increasing joint compression, and reducing strength potential. This pulls the starting point toward the concentric end of the spectrum and the muscles soon spend much more time exploring that end than the opposite; this reinforces imbalance.

The Muscle Contraction Spectrum

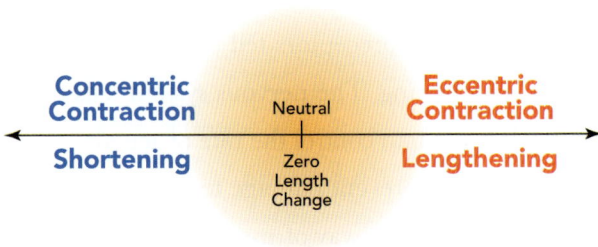

Recently, the approaches to strength training, physical therapy, and sports rehabilitation have focused primarily on loading the shortening, concentric contraction of the muscle with little attention paid to the loading, lengthening, eccentric contraction. It is like reading only the even pages of a book; you miss out on half the story. There are obvious

downsides to the concentric-focused approach. As bones move away from one another the muscles receive length and a greater potential for contraction. As bones move toward each other the muscles shorten. If the bones do not move through their entire range and only stop halfway, the movement and performance potential is much less. If the body doesn't experience muscle contractions at their lengthened end range, the nervous system never gets to experience it either, and may not know what to do when it finds itself in such situations. Therefore, the ability to manage mass and momentum could be greatly affected and diminished.

RULE #2. JOINTS ACT, MUSCLES REACT

A joint is simply the space between where two bones come together. There are 360 joints in the body. Each joint is surrounded by muscles and soft tissue. When the joint moves, it affects the length and tension of the surrounding tissue. Bones that move away from each other will cause the connecting tissue to lengthen. Bones that move toward each other cause the tissue to shorten. When the body is in motion, it is the joint that moves first, followed by a muscular reaction. An example would be sitting down in a chair. Gravity pulls the body downward and the joints must first move in order for this to occur. The muscles do not act first and pull the body into the chair, gravity does that. Muscles react to the joint motion by contracting as they lengthen to slow the body's descent into the chair. Every movement is, in essence, a controlled fall, which is followed by a muscular reaction against gravity. Walking, running, climbing stairs, and even getting off the ground all must first be initiated by gravity and joint motion before the muscles react to move the body further against gravity.

This means that if a joint is not moving correctly, the surrounding muscles and soft tissues do not respond in the way they should. It is by encouraging the joints to move in all three dimensions, with the least amount of restriction, that the muscles and soft tissue will be continually reminded of the role they play in motion. Use it or lose it.

RULE #3. EVERYTHING REVOLVES
AROUND CENTER

Stand still for a moment and close your eyes. Can you feel how your body is constantly managing its mass as it orbits around your center? If you can't, then stand on one leg with your eyes closed and you will sense it instantly. The body is never truly still. Just the subtleties of breathing cause the ribs to expand, the internal organs move to make room for the inflating lungs and dropping diaphragm, and the mass of the body shifts. The nervous system is receiving, interpreting, and sending continual messages to the muscles to contract in such a way that the mass of the body stays above the feet. If that did not happen you would need to take a step to catch yourself, or you would fall down.

As joints move away from a central, balanced position, some muscles must lengthen to allow the bones to move in that direction. However, as some muscles experience lengthening, others must experience shortening. As an example, stand with your feet parallel below the hips. Slowly glide the hips to the left and beyond the left foot. Can you experience the muscles along the left side of the hips getting longer and how they are contracting to keep you from falling over? Did the muscles pull you to the left or did they control your fall? As you return to center can you experience how the same muscles must contract more and shorten to bring you back? This is the essence of human motion.

This constant system of mass management is affected by how the body adapts to its environment and what it experiences. No matter where the body determines where center is, it will constantly attempt to maintain an orbit around that center.

RULE #4. PERCEIVED CENTER DICTATES POSTURE, PERFORMANCE, AND POTENTIAL

When the body is in a balanced, central position, the muscles and joints would be considered at neutral. When the body is at this central location, muscles and joints have the ability to travel equally in either direction. This structural positioning is primarily governed by the subconscious part of the brain. The conscious mind—the frontal lobe and motor cortex—can provide temporary assistance, but ultimately the responsibility resides in the subconscious. A person can consciously stand tall and attempt to find the ideal, proper posture. But remember, there are 206 bones, 360 joints, and 635 muscles to control. It is virtually impossible to consciously control all of that and move from point A to point B. Thus, it is the "old brain," the part of the brain which existed before conscious thought evolved, which determines where the body's center is.

The further away from center the body exists, the less potential it has with regard to muscular force, range of motion, and overall physical performance. Consider Leonardo da Vinci's famous illustration of the Vitruvian Man. The circle that surrounds him marks the outer edge that a person may reach freely. Imagine, instead of a circle, that there is a three-dimensional, oblong shape similar to a watermelon. If a person were to reach in any direction as far as possible without taking more than one step, they would contact the edge of the "watermelon" and experience their potential.

As movement is compromised that watermelon shape shrinks in different areas, closing inward, trapping the body and reducing its potential. Over time, mobility will be further compromised and the human structure will weaken. The sphere will continue to shrink and take away more freedom of movement. Muscles that are too long will not have the capacity to properly shorten back to a normal resting length. Muscles that are too short will have difficulty lengthening back to a normal resting length. Neither scenario is ideal. Over time, if this position is reinforced, the length of the muscles become normalized, the imbalances are maintained, and the joints reside in a compromised, weakened state. The ability to decelerate force wanes.

At one time, this growing inability to decelerate force was observed mostly in seniors and the elderly. Now it can be seen in younger and younger people. Most people have a preferred leg with which they step first when descending a set of stairs. They do not necessarily stop and think which leg should take the first step, it just happens. The pattern gets reinforced the more it happens. It becomes so apparent that many cannot lower themselves with the opposite leg and must take every step down stairs leading with the same side. They are not able to perform the task evenly and their movement potential is diminished while their potential for injury is increased. They have shifted their center of mass so far over to one side that they never get to explore the opposite side in the same way. Watch a person walk bent over a cane, or a person who has an obvious limp or is experiencing back pain or another physical impairment. It is easy to see how their sphere of movement has clamped down upon them, limiting their potential.

RULE #5. THE BRAIN IS HARDWIRED FOR PERFECTION

The nervous system has one primary goal: survival. It will do everything it can to achieve that goal. If the body experiences an injury, the brain will adjust body motion the best way it can to allow the brain to continue to survive. For instance, if a person develops lower back pain, the brain will alter the body's position to move it away from the pain site. It becomes visibly obvious that the person is in pain. The person may lean forward and off to one side. The shoulders may elevate to pull the upper body's mass away from the lower back. Circulation diminishes in the extremities and focuses upon the core and brain. Tension builds and range of motion is reduced.

If the pain becomes too great, the brain will continue to do the best it can, and the person may be forced to get off their feet and lie down. The brain does not ignore the signals; rather, it responds in the best way it can in the moment. It moves away from the threat and draws inward. The drawing in creates the fetal position, the ultimate protective posture. Regardless of what state the physical body is in, the nervous system is always finding the best way to survive. The better balanced and the less pain or threat it encounters the more optimally the body's systems will function.

The upside to this is the brain is teachable. This is known as neural plasticity. The brain is always learning and adapting. This means if the body were guided into new movements and positions which required less effort and felt more comfortable with less or no pain, the brain will encourage the new movement more often than what it had grown accustomed to. This is regardless of how long the structure has been off center or how long pain has been experienced. The area of the brain which regulates posture, accuracy, balance, and coordination does not understand the concept of time. It lives in the moment and simply receives, interprets, and reacts to the stimuli it encounters in that moment. If it is new stimuli that it finds benefit in, it will latch on and want more. This means that just because someone has had low back pain for three months or ten years, they do not have to live with it. We have seen many clients who suffered with chronic pain for decades find relief when their body learns how to return closer to center.

THE FEET

Each foot has 26 bones, 33 joints, and more than 100 muscles, tendons, and ligaments. Every single one of these components is designed to move. Every foot bone is shaped in such a way that when they come together, they create a jigsaw-puzzle-like form. The pieces lock and unlock depending what shape the foot takes, where the weight above is driven down into the foot, and the surface it is landing on. When you step, each of the 26 bones moves in a predetermined timing pattern. This timing pattern enables your foot to absorb the impact, to support weight, and to transfer force into the ground and up through the rest of the body. The force will travel with the least amount of resistance when all the bones, and their corresponding joints, move the way they were evolved to do. In order for the force to flow unimpeded, it is imperative that the foot/ankle complex move in the proper way at the proper time. The same can be said for the knees, hips, pelvis, and so on. Everything balances upon the foot. If the shape of the foot is off center, that has a direct effect on the structures above.

Picture a newly constructed house,

nicely painted, and with a beautifully landscaped yard with a giant oak tree out front. As some time passes, the roots of the oak tree creep under the foundation of the house. The roots grow thick and begin pushing up the foundation at one corner. The structure of the house begins to shift subtly. The walls begin to lean ever so slightly by fractions of an inch. The owner of the house notices one day that the window in the kitchen sticks as it opens. Thinking the wood has gotten wet and has swollen, the owner removes the window, shaves one side with a wood plane,

> **Most athletic movements are directly dependent upon the quality of a person's gait pattern. If the pattern does not occur in the proper sequence, that is when problems have a way of arising.**

and places the window back in the frame. Now it glides smooth and easy with plenty of room. Problem solved. A year later the owner notices the window is sticky again and solves the problem with the same approach. The next year the same thing happens but the owner has shaved so much off the sides of the window that there is nothing more to shave. Time to replace the entire window. Is the problem really the window? No, it is the foundation, which affects the entire house. The sticky window was merely a symptom of the structural imbalance.

POSTURE ASSESSMENT

You will get a greater insight into the position and spacing of your joints, where muscles are too long and too short, and where stress or strain is occurring if you first develop a better understanding of where your body is in space. Take the following assessment. When performing this assessment, you may benefit by standing in front of a mirror to get an "outsider's" perspective of where your body rests in space and where it is moving away from center. For most, the deviations will be subtle and almost unnoticeable. It is something we take for granted and do not pay much attention to.

Take your time and really observe how your body positions itself against gravity. The areas of the body you will "interview" are the feet, knees, hips and pelvis, spine, head, and shoulders. Take a few minutes and answer the questions below. Take notes about what you see and what you feel. To aid you, create a stick figure that represents your posture from a front or rear view as well as a profile.

Illustration of Posture Assessment

FEET

Are they neutral and point straight ahead?

Does one foot turn in or out?

Do both feet turn out?

Does one or both feet turn in?

Do the toes curl under or are they spread out?

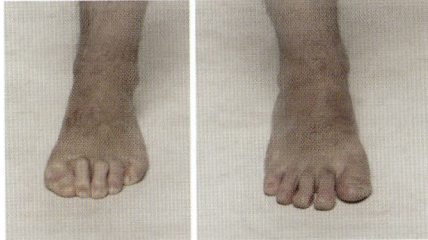

MEDIAL ARCHES

Do the feet have high arches or flat arches?

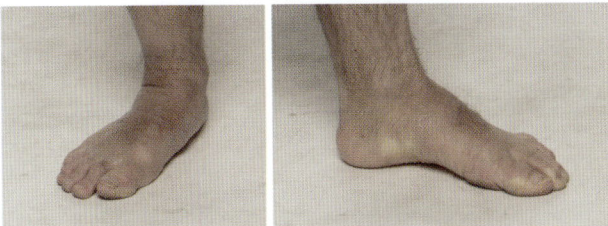

Is one foot flatter?

KNEES

Which knee is more flexed (bent)?

Does one knee hyperextend (go beyond a straight line)?

Is there any rotation at the knees?

Do the knees point in the same direction as the feet?

HIPS & PELVIS

Is the pelvis tilted forward or backward?

Is one side tilted more forward? Left or right?

Is one side of the pelvis higher? Left or right?

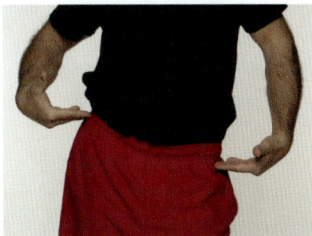

Does the pelvis rotate to the left or right?

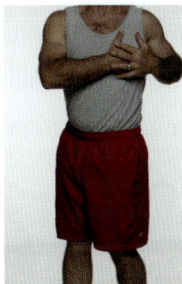

Are the hips more over one leg? Left or right?

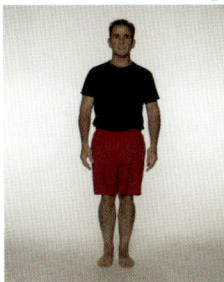

RIBS & SPINE

Are the ribs tilted forward or backward?

Are the ribs shifted to the left or right?

Are the ribs side-bending to the left or right?

Are the ribs rotated to the left or right?

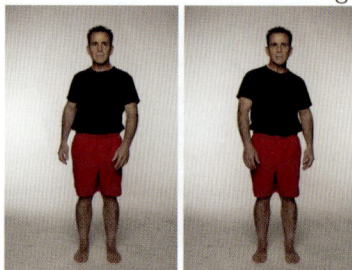

What shape does the spine take?

Is it curved or straight?

Does the spine bend to one side?

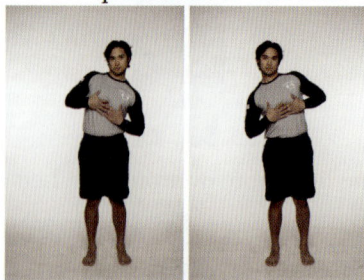

Is the spine rotating to the left or right?

SHOULDERS

Is one shoulder higher? Left or right?

Is one arm rotated in more? Left or right?

Is one shoulder more forward? Left or right?

HEAD

Is the head shifting forward or pulling back?

Is the head tilted forward or backward?

Is the head side-bending to the left or right?

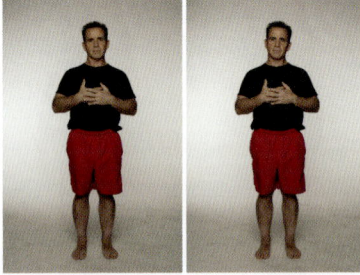

Is the head shifted to the left or right?

Is the head rotated to the left or right?

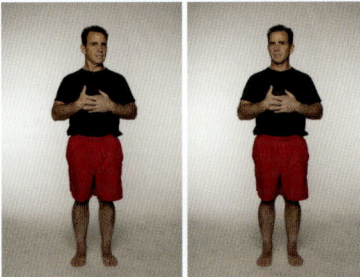

TARGET THE PROBLEM, NOT THE SYMPTOM: SCOLIOSIS

A man in his mid-forties came to see me. He had been suffering from chronic lower back pain and severe scoliosis. While searching on the internet for information about exercise and scoliosis, he came upon an article that had been published a few years back and which featured an interview with me. The topic was what someone could do to help reduce the onset of scoliosis.

He had tried an endless list of approaches to address his spinal contortion. He had seen a spine specialist who put him in a back brace for a couple of years, only to have his supporting muscles atrophy and cause more distortion. He tried an assortment of doctors, physical therapists, and stretching, but nothing had long-lasting effects. Nor had anything been able to alleviate his low back pain, other than prescription medication. In the end, he was told to "work on his core" and that it was only a matter of time before he would need surgery and a hip replacement. He said that seeing me was his last resort.

We sat and talked about his health history to see what might have contributed to his change in posture. He had been diagnosed with scoliosis more than 30 years earlier in middle school. Since he was not born with scoliosis, it makes sense that something must have occurred for his body to change shape, possibly something like trying to avoid pain or discomfort, which ironically and inevitably led to more pain and discomfort. The spine didn't just wake up one day and decide to twist and bend for no reason.

He explained that he had never broken any bones or sprained any joints. When I asked about surgeries, he said he had torn the meniscus in his knee a few years ago and got it repaired. He also said it was the second time that the meniscus had torn. The first time was in high school. Both of these events occurred after his scoliosis diagnosis, so those were ruled out as contributing factors. If anything, the scoliosis might have contributed to the meniscus tears, not the other way around.

I asked him if there were any other surgeries, and he replied he had a hernia repaired when he was five or six years old. Now that was significant! We know a scar will pull surrounding tissue toward its center in an attempt to further close what was, in his case, surgically opened. We also know that when the body encounters pain, it attempts to find the best way to avoid it. Even though the hernia repair was 40 years in the past, if the nerves had not fully reconnected, how would the brain know that the wound had fully healed? Have you ever had a scar where the nerve sensation never fully returns? What might happen if he were to provide some stimuli to let the brain know the scar had healed? I had him place his fingers on the hernia scar and stand up from his seated position. I asked him if he noticed a difference when he stood. He answered that his back didn't pinch like it normally did when he got up. I do not know why touching a scar can have such an effect, but I have witnessed it too many times for it to be disregarded. Imagine yourself at age 5 or 6, just exiting the toddler phase of life, while your bones are still fusing, and walking is still a relatively new challenge. What effect would severing nerves, skin, and muscle tissue have on how you move, carry your weight, and support your structure? Is it too far-fetched to consider? It is not out of the question that, after going through hernia repair, the body would shift away from the affected area and create a new strategy for movement. The pelvis might tilt to one side as the weight shifted away from center. The ribs and spine might have to adjust by side bending, or sheering, to bring mass back over the pelvis. Within the span of seven years, this type of compensatory, post-operative movement developed a scoliotic shift. He had no physical therapy after the operation to help restore proper motion (currently that is still not considered necessary after hernia repairs). Therefore, whatever subconscious way the body chose to organize itself around the affected area, it then reinforced the change to a greater degree. Over the next 30 years, the scoliosis increased because gravity never stopped and no intervention effectively corrected the distortion.

Long story short, we found certain movements in his gait pattern that he was missing and we began to let his body experience them. By balancing the movements that orbit his center we were able to bring about a more balanced structure. Within one session, he was able to stand up without his lower back giving him trouble. When the session was over, the constant, stabbing pain in his low back was gone. The pain had diminished to a dull ache. This was the first time in a very long time that his back had felt so good. The scoliotic spine had also changed a little and he felt his weight shifting away from the areas that were very compressed.

CHAPTER 3
GAIT & DYNAMIC ASSESSMENT

GAIT

If the average American takes 5,000 steps a day, in one year that's 1,825,000 steps. Is there any other movement that we perform with a higher frequency? That is a lot of time on one leg or the other. But, did you know that up to 90 percent of our upright time is spent supporting the body mainly on one leg, and only 10 percent is spent on both legs at the same time? So, why is 90 percent of a strength training routine focused on training the body how it functions only 10 percent of the time (bilaterally)?

Walking is the most universal action that almost every person on Earth performs. This pattern of ambulation has evolved over two million years, which means the nervous system, joints, and muscles (the entire body actually) have developed and cemented amazing relationships with each other to support walking. There is an amazing timing pattern amongst all of the 360 joints of the body as we walk. These relationships are hardwired into our neurological system. They have evolved to be the strongest and most efficient way for moving the entire body. The simple act of walking aids in promoting proper function to every system in the body. Most athletic movements are directly dependent upon the quality of a person's gait pattern. If the pattern does not occur in the proper sequence, that is when problems have a way of arising. If the basic action of walking is compromised, how can a person expect to have efficient athletic actions? You must be able to walk before you can run or jump.

Humans are considered contralateral bipeds. This means we walk on two feet and that the sides of the body move in opposition. Opposition is the name of the game. One leg moves almost exactly opposite to the other. As one leg travels back, the other travels forward. As one begins to load the body's weight on it, the other begins to unload. As one arm swings forward, the other swings back. Opposition also occurs between the pelvis and rib cage. As one tilts forward, the other tilts back. When the pelvis tilts to the left, the ribs tilt right. When one rotates left, the other goes right. This also occurs with the arms. Although the timing does not exactly coincide with the swinging of the legs, the oppositional action is just the same. One arm swings forward, and externally rotates as the elbow flexes, while the other arm swings back, internally rotates, and extends the elbow.

> Every joint should be able to move through three-dimensional space, to its end range, before changing directions and traveling through center on its way to its opposite end range.

The hips and shoulders should experience flexion, extension, abduction, adduction, as well as internal and external rotation.

In fact, every joint should experience all of its ranges of motion in three-dimensional space when we walk. This means that the surrounding muscles and soft tissue experience lengthening, shortening, loading and unloading, tension and compression, in all three dimensions. The more we explore gait mechanics the more we will observe these oppositional actions and other relationships. As the spine flexes, the pelvis should move a certain way. As the arms swing, the shoulder blades, ankles, and jaw should move certain ways. As the knee extends, the neck, wrist, and big toes should move in certain ways. It is all connected. Change one thing, and everything changes.

THE GAIT CYCLE

Gait is viewed as a continuous, cyclical action. One complete gait cycle begins with one heel striking the ground and ends when the same heel strikes again. The cycle can be broken up into specific moments in time like a freeze frame. These freeze frames are called phases. Gait phases occur in one of two categories: swing or stance. Swing refers to when only one foot is in contact with the ground. Stance occurs when both feet are in contact. Gait can be divided into countless moments in the cycle, but the most discernible joint actions occur at the phases. With each phase in the gait cycle comes a complex relationship between every joint. Although the gait cycle occurs in less than one second, the body goes through almost every joint function imaginable.

Anatomy in Motion's *Flow Motion Model®* details every joint action in three dimensions through the entire gait cycle. Normally, fitness professionals, physical therapists, osteopaths, athletic trainers, bodyworkers, chiropractors, and a handful of medical doctors will spend six days in an immersion course to begin to learn all of the actions in a gait cycle, and that is just to get the basic information. It would be too daunting a task to write it all out in these pages. Instead, we will take a general overview in understanding gait.

Rather than dive headfirst into the incredibly complex depth of how 360 joints move in three-dimensional space in the span of less than one second, let us simply cover the basic joint motions and the relationships joints have with other joints of the body. It is by getting these relationships better established that the body will become more efficient, stronger, pliable, and powerful with every movement. If some of these movements are challenging to perform, or feel completely foreign, that lets a person know what might be missing and needs to be reintroduced.

Can the rib cage tilt equally forward and back? Can the rib cage side-bend left as effortlessly as it side-bends right? Does the rib cage rotate left the same way it rotates right? Ask the same questions of the pelvis and the skull. It is this information that will provide great insight to what needs to be improved for improving overall performance. Can the hip flex as well as extend? Can the hips abduct and adduct with little difference? What is the quality of hip rotation on the left compared to the right? Every joint should be able to move through three-dimensional space to its end range before changing directions and traveling through center on its way to its opposite end range. If one movement is limited or unable to occur, where is the compensation? It will appear somewhere within the gait pattern. Unless corrected, the compensatory pattern will continue and the likelihood of future injuries and stress will increase.

The body does not move in isolation, but rather as a closed, integrative unit. When one joint moves in one direction, the rest of the joints in the body respond with their own movements. This does not occur in one simple direction, but in all three dimensions. One action creates a chain reaction. For instance, as the stepping leg fully contacts the ground and weight is being transferred upon it, the pelvis tilts forward, the knee flexes, the ankle flexes, and the arches in the weight-bearing foot drop. Above the pelvis we should witness the spine extending, the neck flexing, the ribs tilting back, and the skull tilting forward. Then there are the lateral actions of the joints at the same moment in time.

> During the 0.6-0.8 seconds it takes to complete the gait cycle, if any joint is not beginning from a central, balanced location, it will not have enough time to travel through the complete journey from one end range to the other. This is when compensation will arise. It will occur throughout the entire system, not just isolated at one joint.

We should witness the pelvis tilting sideways so the higher side is over the leg beginning to bear weight. The hip of the forward leg will adduct, the knee will drive inward, the heel will evert, and the forefoot will invert. Above the pelvis we see the spine laterally flexing (side-bending) in the direction of the forward leg, the ribs going in the same direction of the spine, and the skull tilting away like the pelvis itself. At the same instance, in regard to rotational action, we will see the pelvis rotating away from the forward leg, the hip externally rotating, the knee externally rotating, and the foot/ankle complex internally rotating as the front portion of the foot is externally rotating. Above the pelvis we will see the spine and rib cage rotating toward the forward leg, and the skull rotating away with the pelvis.

In order for the other leg to perform the same action, all of the joint motions listed above have to reach an end point, stop, reverse directions, and travel back through CENTER and on to the other end point. This is just one part of the gait cycle. There are many more motions that occur in certain combinations, at specific moments in gait, and which are paired with specific joint actions elsewhere. This symphony of joint actions, combined with muscular reactions, should occur every time, over and over, for 1.8 million steps per year. This must all occur in the span of less than one second, the time it takes for one full gait cycle to occur. During the 0.6-0.8 seconds it takes to complete the gait cycle, if any joint is not beginning from a central, balanced location, it will not have enough time to travel through the complete journey from one end range to the other. This is when compensation will arise. It will occur throughout the entire system, not just isolated at one joint.

PLAYING THE PERCENTAGES

Here is a simple word problem: There are ten people in a group. Each person holds a fruit basket with six apples in each, for a total of 60 apples. When they are told to begin, each person places an apple in someone else's basket. They continue doing this for five minutes. When the group stops, how many apples do they have in total? The answer is 60. Some might have more apples in their basket and others may have fewer, but the total still remains 60. No apples were lost nor gained. The same can be said of human movement and energy.

Each joint in the body has an ideal amount of movement and force production for which it is responsible at any given time. Similar to the word problem, total joint movement always adds up to a certain amount of movement for someone to travel from point A to point B. Let's just use 100 percent for the sake of argument. Each joint, and its surrounding muscles, should have a certain percentage of participation and amount of force to produce. The bigger joints, like the hips, shoulders, and ankles, typically would have a greater percentage. Meanwhile, the spine, hands, and toes would have a smaller percentage. What would happen if one of the joints reduced its percentage of movement and did not produce as much force? Some other joints would need to increase their movement percentages and the neighboring muscles would need to increase force production. This could happen due to injury, surgery, lack of movement, or a myriad of other physical, hormonal, or emotional elements.

The body would still need to achieve 100 percent of movement and force production. Somewhere else in the body would need to compensate and increase its percentage of movement to get the total to 100 percent. Most times, the shifting of percentages is subtle, but other times it appears quite obvious, such as when someone limps. If the altered pattern of compensatory movement is continually reinforced, many reactions will take place: muscular imbalances, postural distortion, compromised gait patterns, joint and soft tissue wear and inflammation, as well as hormonal and organic stress. Regardless of the degree of percentage altering, the closer a person can achieve ideal joint motion and reduce compensatory patterns, the less likely is the chance of injury.

It is quite common for an individual to have restriction around joints that are inflamed or in the muscles that surround these joints. The limitations can originate in the joints or in the muscles and soft tissues. They feed into one another in a "chicken or egg" sort of way. For instance, chest muscles that are too short restrict joint motions of the shoulders, ribs, and mid-back and will often demand a higher degree of motion from other joints nearby (such as the elbows, wrists, and neck). Hamstring muscles, if too long or shortened, will restrict joint motion of the pelvis, hips, and knees, and demand a higher degree of motion from neighboring joints (such as the knees, ankles, and vertebrae of the low back). Calf muscles that are too long or too short will limit ankle motion and demand more from the neighboring knees or feet. The compensations do not just occur at neighboring joints, but have the potential of occurring anywhere in the body. Sometimes they occur in the most obscure places, as you will continue to read throughout this book.

Now, imagine what it would mean if a joint were to have zero movement. A person subconsciously compensates for restriction in one area of the body only to have another area move more than it should. This might cause such a degree of wear and tear at the place of compensation that surgical fusion is recommended. For example, in spinal fusion, the surgeon takes bone from the pelvis or a cadaver and places it between two or more vertebra to fuse them together. The affected area has been worn down so much from improper movement, that now the opposite solution is prescribed: immobility. All or nothing. Instead of a high percentage of participation, there is now 0 percent. What would you predict would happen next? Remember, total movement still needs to reach 100 percent no matter what. Perhaps you will begin to see the neighboring joints above and below the fusion take on a greater percentage of movement? Or, if the compensatory movement patterns are not addressed, perhaps the fusion breaks apart from continued force in that region? If either occur, it will not be long before another fusion is recommended.

The trouble with this problem-solving approach of using fusion is that, at no point in time does anyone take a step back and look at how the entire body is organizing movement and what each joint's participation percentage is. Do you think that, if that is taken into consideration the powers that be might determine a different course of action? Perhaps they might discover that a restriction in the person's right knee is limiting the range of motion in the hip and causing the spine to compensate enormously? Or perhaps it is the history of shoulder dislocations that

restricted tissue length around the shoulder blade and asked the spine to move more? Or maybe it stems from the whiplash suffered in a car accident that occurred 15 years ago and that forced the lower back to take up the slack of the injured neck? Really, there are an infinite number of possibilities which could occur and then ask the body to adapt and compensate. Determining how the body moves, then encouraging and guiding it

to move in a more efficient and proper manner, might reduce the wearing down of areas that do not deserve such punishment.

Whether you are a top-level athlete, a weekend warrior, or a full-time desk jockey, you will perform at your best when you begin from a balanced, central position. Think of a golfer. Before a golfer swings at the ball, he or she should have an even distribution of weight between both feet. As the club travels back, the body rotates fluidly in a timed sequence and the weight migrates more over the back leg. At the end range of the back swing, the hips begin to rotate in the opposite direction. The rest of the body follows and weight eventually migrates over to the other leg. Now, imagine if the golfer were subtly and unknowingly over one leg

As long as the body is fighting gravity, it will always do its best to keep its mass over the feet.

more than the other prior to the swing. How would that affect the swing mechanics and how the ball is hit?

If a carpenter spends his entire week framing a house in a crouched position with a nail gun, how might that affect his basketball game with his buddies on Saturday morning? If the desk jockey commutes and works a total of 50 hours a week, sitting in the most ergonomically designed car and work station, how will his or her body respond to hauling bags of groceries out of the trunk or getting on the floor to play with the kids after work? Might we expect to see aches and pains develop eventually? Could sprains and strains be a logical forecast? Might the golfer, carpenter, or desk jockey begin to complain of lower back pain or some other joint or muscle issue? If the pain persists, how might that affect the pursuit of what they so enjoy? If they are active gym goers, how might these issues begin to affect their workout? Would they be forced to paint themselves into corners and limit the activities they had been enjoying? Would the exercises they practice in their workout be helping solve the issues or would they be exacerbating them?

What about every time someone simply moves? You see it all the time, but might not stop to consider the long-term effects. You could be sitting on a park bench watching joggers pass by and notice several of them leaning forward more than they should, or one heel kicking back more, or one arm swinging more than the other. You could be watching Grandpa coming down the stairs and notice that he always leads with his left leg when traveling to the next step. You might be walking along the city street and notice someone walking toward you and who looks to be in obvious pain. Their body is shifted to one side or they are limping a bit. Then there are those individuals who do not appear to be moving in a compromised manner. Often, they are the high-level athletes who have learned strategies to get around their limitations. This just means they are good at hiding their faults. If these postures and patterns of movement continue over the course of months or years what might you expect to see? Would some joints begin to get inflamed? Would some muscles be overworked while others are underworked? Would the potential for pain, injury, and surgery increase? Yes! Yes! and Yes!

Unfortunately, for those who are under forty years of age and who exercise regularly, the negative effects of this traditional style of strength training will, most likely, not manifest as pain or injury for many years to come. Perhaps this is why we are seeing an explosion of high-intensity training programs appear in the fitness industry even as the nation continues to become more sedentary, overweight, and de-conditioned. These high-intensity exercisers will experience the positive effects much sooner and that will just reinforce their approach all the more. It takes time for the body to wear down. Perhaps there will be just little nagging aches to start. They will change or modify their exercises to avoid the pain, but their training programs will continue to draw them off their center.

EIGHT BODY SHAPES

Even though the body can be contorted into a variety of positions, there are certain limitations and only so many ways the body can move. We live in three dimensions. We can travel forward and back, side to side, up and down, and turn left and right. This pertains to the whole body and the parts it is made up of, such as the pelvis, skull, spine, etc. There are only so many directions the pelvis can move: shift left or right, up or down, forward or back, or spin left or right. Many combinations of these basic actions can be achieved. Rather than being a one-dimensional motion, it is often multidimensional. This is how our bodies move. This is how we walk. It is a combination of three-dimensional motions. As long as

the body is fighting gravity, it will always do its best to keep its mass over the feet. It does so by shifting different areas in different directions at varying times. If too much mass travels outside of this area (known as the base of support), there are two options: take a step and reposition the mass above the feet, or fall down. Think of a circus performer who balances a pole in the palm of their hand as a plate spins at the top. The performer is constantly adjusting the hand position in order to keep everything balanced and the plate from falling.

To better understand these combinations of multidimensional movement, let us look at each individual dimension of motion at a time and how the body manages its mass as it moves. These motions should naturally occur when everything is in its proper, balanced place and is unrestricted. The dimensions of movement are known as *planes of motion*. The *sagittal plane of motion* applies to forward and backward action. The *frontal (or coronal) plane* applies to lateral or sideways action. The *transverse plane* applies to rotational action. We see that when one area travels in one direction, another part of the body travels in the opposite. This is how muscles lengthen and shorten, how joints open and close. It is by oppositional motion that we travel through the world. When we separate each dimensional movement in the planes of motion, as they relate to the gait cycle, we find a total of eight basic shapes. These are the motions that should naturally occur when walking and running. Provided the body achieves all eight positions, movement is at its most optimal.

The patterns of compensation a person develops are as unique as their fingerprints.

TWO SAGITTAL PLANE POSITIONS

In Figure 1, the pelvis tilts anteriorly (forward) while the ribs tilt posteriorly (backward) and the thoracic and lumbar spine is extending. Can you imagine how the abdominals, gluteals, and hamstrings must lengthen while the hip flexors, quadriceps, and lower back muscles shorten? The skull (although level with the ground) must tilt anteriorly like the pelvis if it is to stay balanced over the posteriorly tilting rib cage. Can you get a sense of how the muscles along the back of the neck must lengthen while the front shortens? If we were to bring in other parts of the body, we would see the shoulders and scapulae (shoulder blades) retract back and down toward the spine. This would encourage the pectorals (chest muscles) and upper trapezius to lengthen while the rhomboids and middle and lower trapezius muscles shortened. We would see the hips and knees move into flexion while the ankle dorsiflexes and the feet journey into pronation.

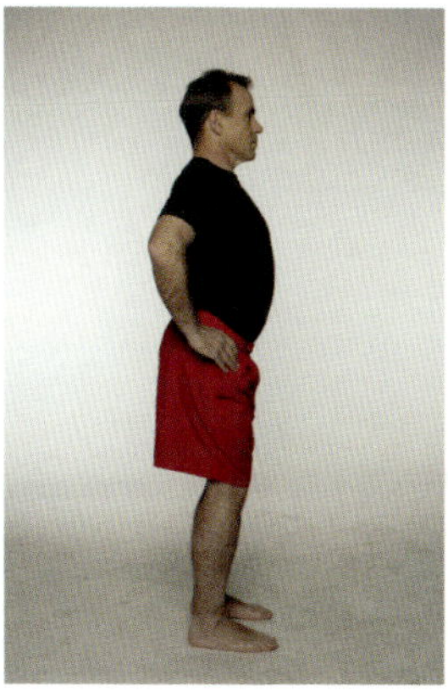

FIGURE 1 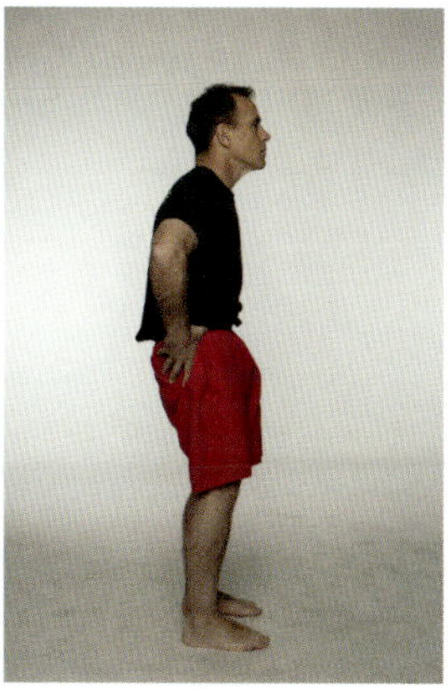   FIGURE 2

In Figure 2, the movement is the polar opposite of Figure 1. The pelvis posteriorly tilts as the ribs anteriorly tilt as the spine flexes. The abdominals, gluteals, and hamstrings shorten while the hip flexors, quadriceps, and lower back muscles lengthen. The skull matches the pelvis in its posterior tilt to maintain a level position above the torso. The muscles along the back of the neck shorten as the front of the neck lengthens. Bringing in other parts, we see the shoulders elevate and protract. This would cause the upper trapezius and pectorals to shorten, and the rhomboids, and lower and middle trapezius to lengthen. The hips and knees come out of their flexed position and travel in the opposite direction into extension. The ankles would planter flex as the feet journey into supination.

FOUR FRONTAL PLANE POSITIONS

In Figure 3, you can also see the oppositional relationship of each body segment. The pelvis travels to the left as the rib cage travels right and the skull matches the pelvis. One leg experiences the pelvis moving toward its direction while the other leg experiences it traveling away. Can you get the sense that muscles on the opposite side will have different degrees of length? As one area on the left shortens, the same area on the right must lengthen. Consider the adductor muscles of the inner thighs. As the pelvis travels to the left, the left adductors shorten while the right adductors are forced to lengthen.

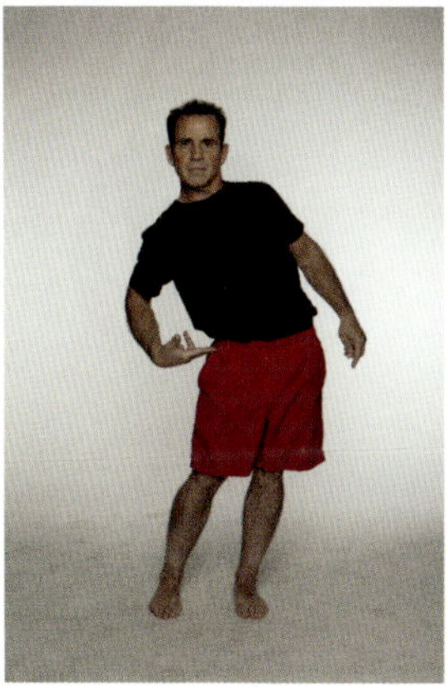

FIGURE 3 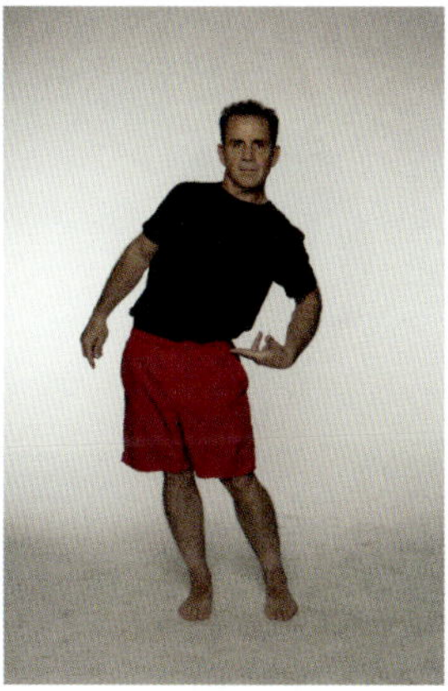   FIGURE 4

Figure 4 is the mirror image of Figure 3. We can travel far to the left and far to the right. The biggest difference between this position and all the others is the body travels off its vertical axis. This means the head is not lined up directly over the rib cage. The ribs are not lined up directly over the pelvis. The pelvis travels away from being above and between both feet. This is the most precarious position the body can find itself in during the gait cycle. All other body positions maintain alignment of the body's mass on the vertical axis.

Figures 5 and 6 demonstrate another way of traveling sideways. Instead of swaying, the action is a lateral tilt. The movement is also along the frontal plane but just in a different manner. The oppositional actions still take place. As the pelvis tilts one direction, the rib cage tilts opposite. As one leg flexes at the knee the other extends. The two types of frontal plane motions are part of how we transfer weight on to one foot and then reverse directions to get the weight over to the other side. They do not occur simultaneously but at different times in the gait cycle. This is important to know, because many will unconsciously create a strategy of motion which encourages one type of frontal plane action over the other.

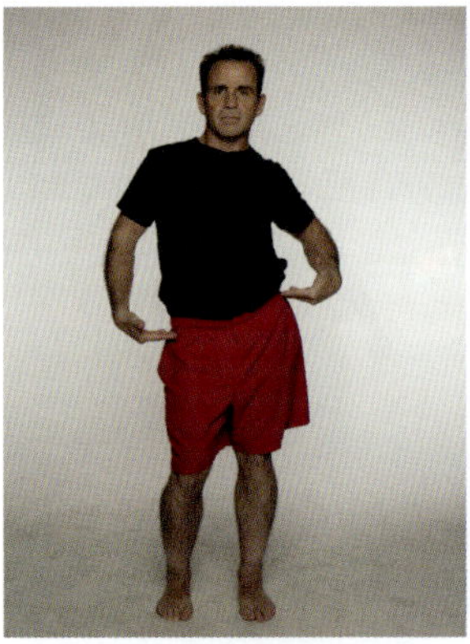

FIGURE 5 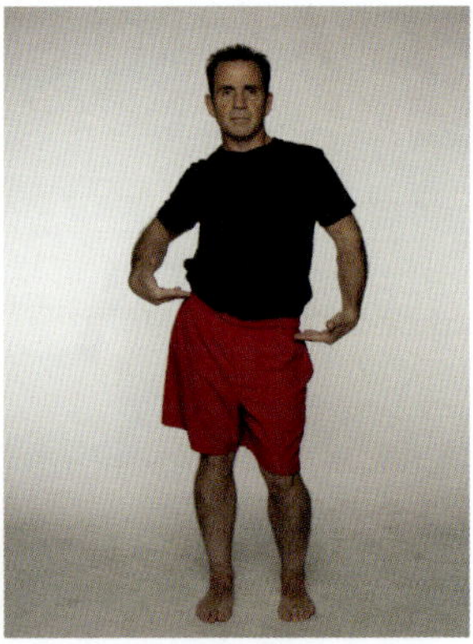   FIGURE 6

TWO TRANSVERSE PLANE POSITIONS

Rotation is a major component of sending the body through space, and Figures 7 and 8 are all about rotation. You can see in Figure 7 how the pelvis rotates left as the rib cage rotates right. With the skull staying balanced and facing forward it is actually rotating opposite of the rib cage. Once again we see the pelvis and skull opposing the action of the rib cage. We can also see opposition between the legs. As the pelvis rotates toward one side, one leg begins internally rotating at the hip while the other externally rotates. The same opposing action occurs with the arms as the rib cage rotates. The feet will also experience opposing actions as one begins to pronate, the other begins to supinate.

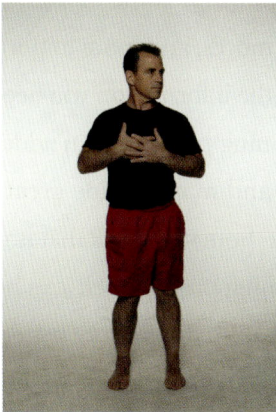 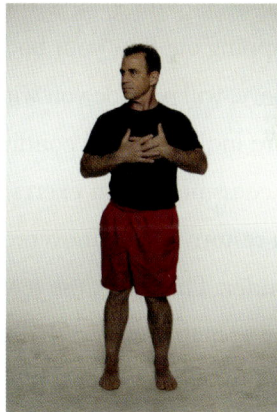

FIGURE 7   FIGURE 8

THE DYNAMIC ASSESSMENT

Have you ever interviewed your body? Can you reach freely and equally in all directions? Do you feel more restricted than you believe you should be? Do you have any imbalances? Do you experience pain or discomfort at any point? Where are the places in your sphere of motion that have shrunken inward? Chances are you already have some awareness of the areas of limitations. Perhaps you are like many others who choose to believe that this is normal and there is not much you can do about it. Chalking it up to just getting older? If these are your truths then let's set to smashing them right now.

This is where you get to find out what patterns have been reinforced and which joint actions are restricted, or for some of you, completely foreign. Mapping out how your body moves, and more importantly, how it doesn't move, will provide you with the information you need to create a much more individualized conditioning program. An added bonus is that every assessment is an exercise and may provide great benefit in helping you restore proper movement. Sometimes, all that is needed is a gentle reminder. Therefore, the screening process itself can be used as a daily routine to help unlock restricted areas and restore better structural balance. You should also use it regularly as your guide to designing the right conditioning routine. It is not just a one-time deal!

The body is designed for optimal movement. The spine needs to be able to flex and extend, tilt left and right, as well as rotate left and right. The hips and shoulders need to be able to flex and extend, adduct and abduct (move toward and away from the body), as well as internally and externally rotate. These are just some of the major movements the body goes through, but there are dozens more that involve the elbows, wrists, hands, knees, ankles, and feet. When one joint moves slower or less than it should, one or more other joints need to speed up or move more. This also occurs in reverse. Everyone has a certain amount of this altering of joint action and it is their subconscious way to compensate. The patterns of compensation a person develops are as unique as their fingerprints. In the short term, these compensatory patterns may be necessary to move with the least amount of pain, and may not be noticeable. However, the continued compensations can bring about wear and tear, inflammation, more pain, and suffering. It is then just a matter of time before the body eventually gets to a point when symptoms begin to appear. It is not so much aging as it is the length of time under compensatory tension and compression.

Remember, the body is always adapting to its environment. Even if you exercise for an hour every day, chances are there are still 161 hours during the week when you are not, and your body adapts to those hours. That could mean the workout you performed last week may not be what your body needs this week. To keep repeating the same workout routine, the same repetitive motions, may not be the best approach. Too often, individuals choose exercises for areas of the body they are already proficient with and thus these areas are overstimulated. People are focusing on the strong links in the chain and not the weak ones. This has a greater chance of reinforcing muscular imbalances, postural distortions, and reduced joint function. When the person gets to the gym it just makes sense that they would gravitate to the places that are already stimulated rather than search for the under-stimulated areas. The brain tends to lose touch with under-stimulated areas and clears those regions off its neural map of the body. The trouble is, people continue doing the same exercises day after day, and week after week, until symptoms of overwork have appeared, such as shoulder impingement when bench pressing or elbow pain when curling the barbell.

It is by understanding your unique ways of moving, and what is missing in your patterns, where you will develop the knowledge of which movements will benefit you. If you find that some of your movements are restricted, difficult, or foreign, those are the movements you may want to address in your conditioning program. This assessment is your ongoing guide! Take the guesswork out of exercise selection and have your body tell you exactly what it needs.

Following are ten movement assessments. These ten movement assessments are comprised of the basic elements of what humans have been doing for two million years, that is, walking on two feet. The movements are taken from the *Flow Motion Model*®, created by Gary Ward. *Flow Motion Model*® is a map of what the entire body must go through when traveling through the gait cycle. Every joint and muscle has a key role to play in literally every step. If the timing is off in one area of the body it throws the timing off everywhere else. That means every movement, every posture, every athletic action is affected. Each joint has a neurological and mechanical relationship with all of the other joints in the body. How can they not? They are all connected to one another.

Imagine a long line of people standing side by side, holding hands. If the person in the middle of the line were to fall, how would that affect the people on the ends? The same may be said of an area where there is no movement. Stagnation occurs. No change of length in the tissue. Reduced circulation and stimulation which often bring about inflammation. Most would call this arthritis. Sure, you could take anti-inflammatories and pain killers, but does that deal with the underlying problem, which is a lack of motion? All joints are designed for movement, so if one does not move well it might be nice to give it the gift of experiencing motion. All the other joints will benefit from the gift as well because that one joint not moving alters how everywhere else moves. You may be amazed that simply by getting a stiff elbow or wrist joint to move better, how much power and balance improves in your daily life.

When you perform each movement assessment, the goal is not to go as far as possible, but to get a sense of the quality of motion in each direction. Is there a difference? Is one direction more natural and the other uncertain? Be subjective. Think of descriptive words such as smooth, creamy, rough, forced, effortless, foreign, or bumpy when describing each motion. Does one direction feel like it is what you need and the other direction is where you commonly find yourself? Be sure to place a checkmark next to the movements that seem to be missing so you can choose from the list of exercises best suited for you.

After completing all of the movements, choose one or two that were the most restricted, or which you feel you need to improve the most. Trust your instincts. If you are unsure, have a friend observe the assessment from an outsider's perspective. Chapters 4, 6, and 7 include a list of mobility drills, strength exercises, and soft tissue targets designed to help address each limitation. It is not necessary to perform every exercise, drill, or target site. Simply choose a few of each to explore and see how the body responds. You do not need to repeat the same exercises at every workout. It would depend on where the restrictions lie in your body. By checking in with how your body moves, and where restrictions are, your workout will be guided by your body's ability rather than an arbitrary selection of movements.

One rule to remember: **Do not move into pain!** If you drive your body into a painful place, the autonomic response known as "fight or flight" kicks in. This protective reflex will cause your body to tighten up and restrict motion. This response also has the capacity to reduce the amount of force a muscle will generate, in essence placing your body in a weakened state. The "no pain, no gain" mentality is counterproductive to the goal of developing a better conditioned body. Pain is your subconscious mind's way of communicating to your conscious mind that something is not correct. The brain is sensing a threat. It is your job to listen and not create more pain.

HOW TO PERFORM THE FOLLOWING ASSESSMENTS:

- Go slowly, very slowly, through each motion.

- Do NOT force the body into an end range of motion.

- Pay attention to the quality of movement more than the quantity or range of motion.

- Be descriptive with words to explain how each motion feels.

- Do NOT move into pain.

- Breathe and relax through each movement.

- If you experience pain, reduce the range of motion until you don't experience pain.

- Pay attention to foreign motion that does not feel natural.

- Pay attention to the difference between each direction of motion or side of the body.

- Make a note of which motions feel like what the body is missing.

THE TEN MOVEMENT ASSESSMENTS

Movement 1:
Anterior (forward) Tilt
Posterior (backward) Tilt

In a standing posture with your feet parallel, begin slowly tilting the pelvis forward as if it were a bowl of water that would pour out of the belly button. Next, begin tilting the pelvis in the opposite direction so the imaginary water pours out the tailbone. Can you perform this motion without sending the hips forward and back? Is there a difference between the directions? Does one feel more natural than the other? If you experience pain, do not go that deep into the movement. If one movement feels like it is what your body needs, or if it is difficult to go one way compared to the other, make a note.

Make a note: What motion do you feel is missing or you struggle to achieve?

Movement 2:
Left Pelvic Sway
Right Pelvic Sway

Stand comfortably with your feet parallel, under the hips. Imagine standing in a very narrow hallway where the chest and thighs touch the wall in front and the buttocks and shoulders touch the wall behind. Slowly sway your hips to the right and then to the left without any rotation or motions forward or back. What is the quality of motion? Is there one direction which the hips fell into and the other direction into which they needed to be driven? Did one side experience a stretch sensation and the other side did not? If one movement feels like it is what your body needs, or if it is difficult to go one way compared to the other, make a note.

Make a note: What motion do you feel is missing or you struggle to achieve?

Movement 3:
Left Hip Hike
Right Hip Hike

Stand comfortably with your feet parallel, under the hips. Slowly bend one knee. Does the same-side hip begin to drop and the opposite-side hip begin to rise? Are you able to do the motion with little or no rotation? Return to the starting position and perform the same knee bend on the opposite leg. What is the quality of this movement? Try to use specific adjectives when describing, rather than just good or bad. Does one cause pain or discomfort? Where does the weight of the body shift when the knee bends? Is it over the straight leg or the bent leg? Does the weight of the body stay only over one leg no matter which knee is bending? If one movement feels like it is what your body needs, or if it was difficult to go one way compared to the other, make a note.

Make a note: What motion do you feel is missing or you struggle to achieve?

Movement 4:
Left Pelvic Rotation
Right Pelvic Rotation

Stand tall with your feet parallel. Keeping the upper body still, slowly rotate the pelvis to the left and then to the right. What is the quality of motion? Is there one direction which the hips fell into and in the other direction did they need to be pushed or pulled into the movement? Did one side experience a stretch the other side did not? How was the rotation created? Did one side do all of the work or was it symmetrical? Was there pain or discomfort? If one movement feels like it is what your body needs, or if it is difficult to go one way compared to the other, make a note.

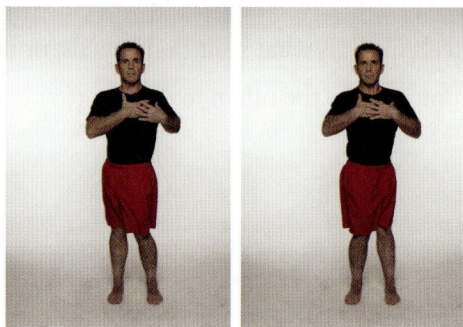

Make a note: What motion do you feel is missing or you struggle to achieve?

Movement 5:
Anterior (forward) Tilt
Posterior (backward) Tilt

In a standing posture with your feet parallel, begin slowly tilting the ribs forward and back. Can you do this without bowing forward or leaning back? Can the tilt occur above the hips? What is the quality of movement between both directions? If one movement feels like it is what the body needs, or if it is difficult to go one way compared to the other, make a note.

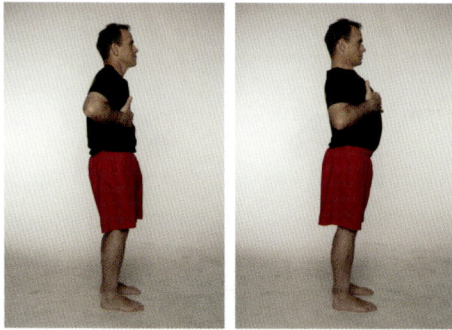

Make a note: What motion do you feel is missing or you struggle to achieve?

Movement 6:
Left Lateral Tilt
Right Lateral Tilt

Stand in a tall posture with your feet parallel. Imagine the axis of rotation is at the sternum (breastbone). Slowly tilt your ribs laterally to the left and then to the right. Were the ribs able to move purely on the axis of rotation? Did the movement occur evenly on both sides? What was the quality of movement? Was there pain or discomfort? If one movement feels like it is what your body needs, or if it is difficult to go one way compared to the other, make a note.

Make a note: What motion do you feel is missing or you struggle to achieve?

Movement 7:
Left Rib Rotation
Right Rib Rotation

Stand tall with your feet parallel. While keeping your lower body still, slowly rotate the ribs to the left and then to the right. What is the quality of motion? Is there one direction which the ribs fell into and the other direction which they needed to be pushed or pulled into? Did one side experience a stretch and the other side did not? How was the rotation created? Did one side do all of the work or was it symmetrical? Was there pain or discomfort? If one movement feels like it is what your body needs, or if it is difficult to go one way compared to the other, make a note.

Make a note: What motion do you feel is missing or you struggle to achieve?

Movement 8:
Left Shoulder Flexion
Right Shoulder Flexion

Stand tall with your feet parallel. Keep the elbows straight and slowly raise one arm at a time forward and overhead. Do not attempt to force the arms upward as high as possible. Instead, only go to the point where resistance is felt (as if you suddenly hit a soft wall and would need even more force to continue). Is there a difference between the arms? What is the quality of movement? Is there any pain or discomfort? If one movement feels like it is what your body needs, or if it is difficult for one arm to go upward compared to the other, make a note.

Make a note: What motion do you feel is missing or you struggle to achieve?

Movement 9:
Left Shoulder Abduction
Right Shoulder Abduction

Stand in a tall posture with your feet parallel. Rotate both palms forward and keep the elbows straight. Slowly raise the arms out to the sides and overhead. Did it occur evenly on both sides? Do not attempt to force the arms upward as high as possible. Instead, only go to the point where resistance is felt (as if you suddenly hit a soft wall and would need even more force to continue). Is there a difference between the arms? What was the quality of movement? Was there pain or discomfort? If one movement feels like it is what your body needs, or if it is difficult to go one way compared to the other, make a note.

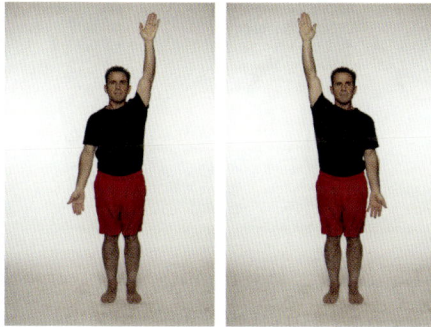

Make a note: What motion do you feel is missing or you struggle to achieve?

Movement 10:
Left and Right Internal Rotation
Left and Right External Rotation

Stand in a tall posture with your feet parallel and with your arms straight. Slowly rotate both palms and arms internally and keep the elbows straight. Reverse directions and rotate the palms and arms externally. Did rotation occur evenly on both sides? Is there a difference between the arms? What was the quality of movement? Was there pain or discomfort? If one movement feels like it is what your body needs, or if it is difficult to go one way compared to the other, make a note.

Make a note: What motion do you feel is missing or you struggle to achieve?

Every joint and muscle has a key role to play in literally every step. If the timing is off in one area of the body it throws the timing off everywhere else.

TARGET THE PROBLEM, NOT THE SYMPTOM: SCARS

Often, scars are easily discounted and no importance is placed upon them. They are thought to be old news with no relevance in the present. Yet, what many may not realize is that scars have the potential to cause trouble somewhere down the road. Not always, but sometimes. To better understand how this might be, consider the function of our skin. What is its primary purpose? It is the largest organ of the body and plays a critical role in our survival. It is part of our immune system. Simply put, it keeps out bad things from getting into our blood stream.

What happens when you get cut? Your insides are exposed to the outside. The depth of the cut determines how much flesh and how many nerve endings get severed. The body's automatic response is to close down on that open area to keep anything from getting in (and keep your blood from getting out). It is a very primitive response to maintain your survival.

What is it that helps close down the area? Clotting occurs to seal the wound. Also staples, sutures, and super glue are modern medical ways to seal the opening. Eventually the cut heals over. However, when the scar forms, the severed nerve endings remain severed and it will take a very long time for sensation across the scar to reoccur, if it ever does. Imagine what the brain is going through during this time of limited nerve sensation. As far as the brain is concerned there is still a hole, because it cannot feel the connection across severed nerve endings.

Your skin and muscles tighten around the area and your posture may change to accommodate the continued protective response. It takes only a short amount of time before this protective response normalizes into your everyday posture. If you have ever undergone surgery, you have probably experienced how scar tissue limits movement. It has become a common approach in the world of physical therapy to try and break up scar tissue to allow the body more freedom of movement. But what if the scar tissue does not break up, what if you have no physical therapy, or what if the nerves never repair themselves? How would the locally restricted movement affect your whole body? What if you were able to bring attention and awareness to the scar area so the brain could get feedback that it is, in fact, healed? Simply touching the scar and getting the body to move could potentially have amazing results.

We had a client some time back who was suffering from low back pain. We went through a health history and learned that he sustained a massive head injury when he was a child. It required major surgery, which left a metal plate under, and a sizable scar across, his forehead. We checked his range of motion at various joints. We found he had significant restrictions that needed to be removed. We guided him through some movements, but the restrictions did not change. Then we had him place his palm over the scar on his forehead, and his range of motion at all of the joints significantly improved. We were able to guide him again through some movements while he held the area of his scar and the result was no more low back pain. It may seem pretty far-fetched, but it happened, nonetheless. His whole posture had reorganized itself around the injury and eventually created an environment for low back pain to occur.

Another client's right shoulder was limited in flexion (she had trouble raising her right arm straight up overhead). She had injured the shoulder when she was aggressively performing a bridge pose in her yoga class. Yet, when we had her touch the scar on her lower back (which she told us was from having a mole surgically removed), she was able to easily enable her right shoulder to travel through the proper range of motion. The scar was over the biggest muscle of the upper body, the latissimus dorsi, which connects the arm to the spine and pelvis. Could it have contributed to restricted shoulder function when she was performing the bridge pose and placed the shoulder in a compromised position? All we know is that when she stimulated the scar area her shoulder function improved.

Is it out of the question to think that a person who underwent a hysterectomy or hernia repair or mastectomy may develop low back pain, elbow tendinitis, or other joint pain because of being restricted elsewhere in their body? The protective tension surrounding a hysterectomy or hernia repair may lead to a laterally shifted and rotated pelvis. It could also bring about a forward tilting rib cage, which would compromise the spine's position, and which also asks other areas to work harder to overcome the restricted joint mechanics. A mastectomy might draw the same-side shoulder forward and inward as a means of protecting the area, causing limited shoulder function and asking the elbow, neck, or wrist to overwork. Unfortunately, there is little research about scars and their effect on movement and chronic pain.

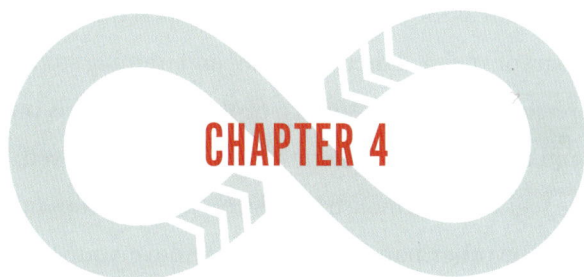

CHAPTER 4

SELF-MYOFASCIAL RELEASE (SMR)

Therapeutic massage has been around for more than 5,000 years. It has been used to heal injuries, relieve pain, and prevent, and possibly, cure illnesses. It is known to reduce stress and produce deep relaxation. There is no need to get into the fine details of how and why this works, just understand that soft tissue work has many benefits. A simple explanation is that when muscle tissue finds itself in a shortened or lengthened state, and returning to its ideal length is not occurring, thus distorting posture, the amount of circulation in the tissue is diminished. Lack of movement decreases circulation. This can apply to a person who is sedentary as well as to a very active individual who has areas of the body that are restricted. We can think about getting the short muscles to become longer and the longer muscles to shorten, but what both also need is better circulation.

This is where Self-Myofascial Release (SMR) comes into play. Most people are now familiar with foam rolling. In fact, this type of SMR work has become so popular that other devices have been created to get those "hard-to-reach" areas. Sticks, balls, peanut-shaped rollers, and canes are an integral part of physical therapy clinics and training studios today. By applying pressure against the surface of the body, fluid is pushed away from the center of pressure. When that pressure is removed, fluid flows back into the region. To demonstrate, place a few fingertips firmly against the back of your other hand. When you remove your fingertips, you should notice a color change on the back of your hand. Did you see the light-colored circles where you had pressed your fingertips begin to fade and become flesh-toned again? You have just created a pumping action of fluid into that area. Areas of the body that have too much tension (length) or too much compression (shortening) also have a reduction of circulation. Often, restoring proper circulation to an affected area will enable better movement and function into the region, which will be able to hydrate itself. Performing soft tissue work on a continual basis may help to maintain a more optimal level of movement and overall performance. The question that needs to be addressed is which areas of the body should you target?

One common and simple strategy many take is to roll out the sore spots; that is, search and destroy. Although this may be effective for some, there is a potential and significant drawback to this approach. Just because an area is sore does not mean it needs to be rolled out. When it comes to tender soft tissue like the IT band (tissue running along the outside of the thigh) or the piriformis muscle (small muscle deep within the buttocks), continually rolling the area of pain might lead to development of more inflammation and tension in the region, further increasing tenderness within the soft tissue. If you continue to roll areas that are tender, over time, the level of tenderness may actually increase. This should be an indicator that rolling that area is not the proper place to target.

A better strategy is to start with a goal of returning the body to a more centered, balanced position. The closer the body gets to the "Goldilocks" spot, the more improved that circulation, muscular balance, joint spacing, and positioning will be, and the less stress that will be applied on the human structure. Therefore,

> Often someone will continue to roll areas that are tender, and over time, the level of tenderness does not change. It may actually increase. This should be an indicator that rolling that area is not the proper place to target.

understanding where the body is positioned over the feet will provide the insight needed to target the proper areas for rolling. Because the body is always changing and adapting to its environment, it is a good idea to always perform a "check in" with how you hold your weight and the position of your structure before each rolling session. You may find that one day you should perform soft tissue hydration along the right inner thigh and the next you will need to target a completely different area. Do not fall into the habit many people do and mindlessly roll the same spots over and over, week after week. The purpose of rolling is to create change and improve movement and function. It is not to beat yourself up by trying to annihilate the sore spots.

In this book, I'm offering you three ways to assess what areas of the body might benefit from foam rolling. The first is using foot pressure as a quick guide. The second is by going through the posture assessment (see Chapter 2) to understand where your structure resides in space and which areas are under tension or compression. The third is performing the ten movement assessments (see Chapter 3) to understand where there is little movement between joints. The assessments will give you a better understanding of not only which strength exercises and mobility drills may benefit you, but also the target areas for rolling.

SEVEN FOOT PRESSURES

There are three arches in each foot. The most well-known of these is the medial arch that runs along the insole from the first metatarsal head (the pad before the big toe) to the calcaneus (heel bone). The second is called the lateral arch, which runs from the fifth metatarsal head (the pad before the small toe) to the calcaneus. The third is called the transverse arch; it runs over the roof of the foot, is formed by the tarsal and metatarsal bones, and is supported by tendons and ligaments. Along with three arches, each foot has three primary points of contact: 1st metatarsal head, 5th metatarsal head, and the calcaneus. These contact points create a tripod of support. When the feet have just the right amount of arch (not too much or little) the three contact points have the proper amount of pressure to distribute body weight and the body is encouraged to be in a more central position. The closer the body is to center, the more efficiently the body functions.

Internal (medial) longitudinal arch

Transverse (or anterior) arch

External (lateral) longitudinal arch

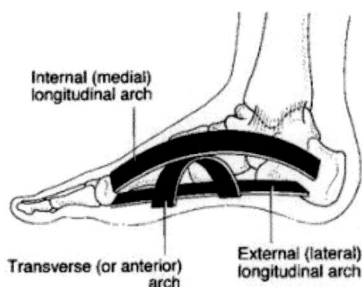

Three arches and the three contact points

Foot shapes will cause the mass of the body to move. Equally so, if the mass of the body shifts, it will cause the shape of the foot to change. Thus, changes in structure and foot shape can come from the top down or from the bottom up. This can place strain in one or more areas, just like the sticky window in the house with an altered foundation.

Much information can be gleaned simply by knowing where pressure is felt on the surface of the feet. If you were to stand with feet parallel and explore how the body travels through each of the eight body positions (see Chapter 3), you would feel how the pressure changes in the soles of the feet. This is also occurring when we stand in our "normal" resting posture. If more of the body's weight is shifted forward or back, to the left or right, there will be a shift in foot pressure. If there is more pressure on one foot, this suggests that there is an imbalance between the left and right side. If more pressure is felt on one heel and the opposite forefoot, that suggests a torque or rotation to the body. If more pressure is experienced in both forefeet, or in both heels, it suggests that a combination of counterbalancing, tilting joints forward and back, exist. Gaining this insight as to where the pressure resides in your feet will give you a better understanding of how you bear your body weight and which areas need to be balanced. Ideally, there should be equal pressure between the left and right foot and fairly equal pressure between the front and back. These four areas (front left and right, and back left and right) should each bear 25 percent of the body's weight.

Where is the pressure of your body weight in your feet? Without wearing shoes and socks, stand on an even surface and see if you can detect where you feel the most pressure. Is there more pressure on one foot compared to the other? Is there more pressure toward the heels or toward the forefeet? Is the pressure greater toward the outside edge of the feet or inside? If you are uncertain where the most pressure is located, then focus on where the least amount of pressure is. This could be equally valuable to understand.

"PRESSURE CHECK IN":

- Remove your shoes.
- Stand in a relaxed, comfortable posture.
- Discern where the most pressure in each foot is felt:
  » Is it more on one foot than the other?
  » Is the pressure more toward the forefoot or toward the heels?
  » Is the pressure more toward the inside or outside of the foot?
  » Is the pressure different on one foot compared to the other?
- If you encounter difficulty feeling where the pressure is, you might try and do the opposite. Where is there the *least* amount of pressure?

As I mentioned earlier, the center of mass for the body should reside equally on the left and right feet. It should also be halfway between the heels and forefeet, and halfway between the inner and outer soles. If all is equal, the foot pressure would then be completely even. Fifty percent left and fifty percent right. This means that each quadrant (left and right forefeet, and left and right heels) should bear 25 percent of the pressure. This is the "Goldilocks" spot. Unfortunately, it is uncommon for anyone in an industrialized nation to find themselves in that position. Over the years the body has subtly shifted some of its mass off center. At our training facility we often have individuals stand on an electronic force plate to gain an idea of how they manage their mass over their feet.

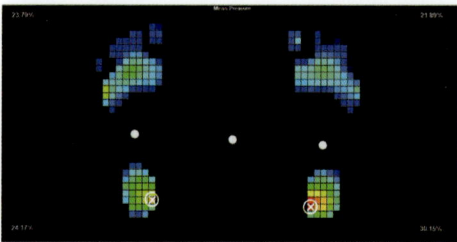

The direction to which the pressure travels is typically where many muscles experience lengthening. The skeletal frame is driving into tissue and causing it to lengthen. Imagine driving your fingers into a latex balloon. The material stretches and lengthens as you drive further into it. The opposite direction is where the muscles will passively shorten because the body is moving away and they naturally take up the slack. Understanding where the body's mass is tending to go will give you a map of where to roll.

So now the question is, which muscles and tissue should you be targeting? The long or the short? For example, if you found that there is more pressure in the front of both feet you could roll the hip flexors and the quadriceps because those areas may very well be longer than they should be. The circulation in that area may be diminished and in need of some rehydration. Or you could target the opposite areas of the gluteus maximus and the hamstrings, as they are in a shortened state and also in need of rehydration via foam rolling. This means that whichever direction the pressure is being directed, you could roll the tissue on that side and its opposite direction. However, over the years we have found the majority of people benefit most by targeting the shortened areas. A smaller percentage get better results when targeting the lengthened areas. This means you have to choose one and then reassess and determine if the rolling brought about the desired result. It is one or the other. It will not take long for your body to inform you. That is why there are two different assessment charts on the following pages. One SMR chart provides a list of lengthened tissue and one of shortened tissue.

FOAM ROLLING TARGETS
SHORTENED TISSUE
BASED ON FOOT PRESSURES

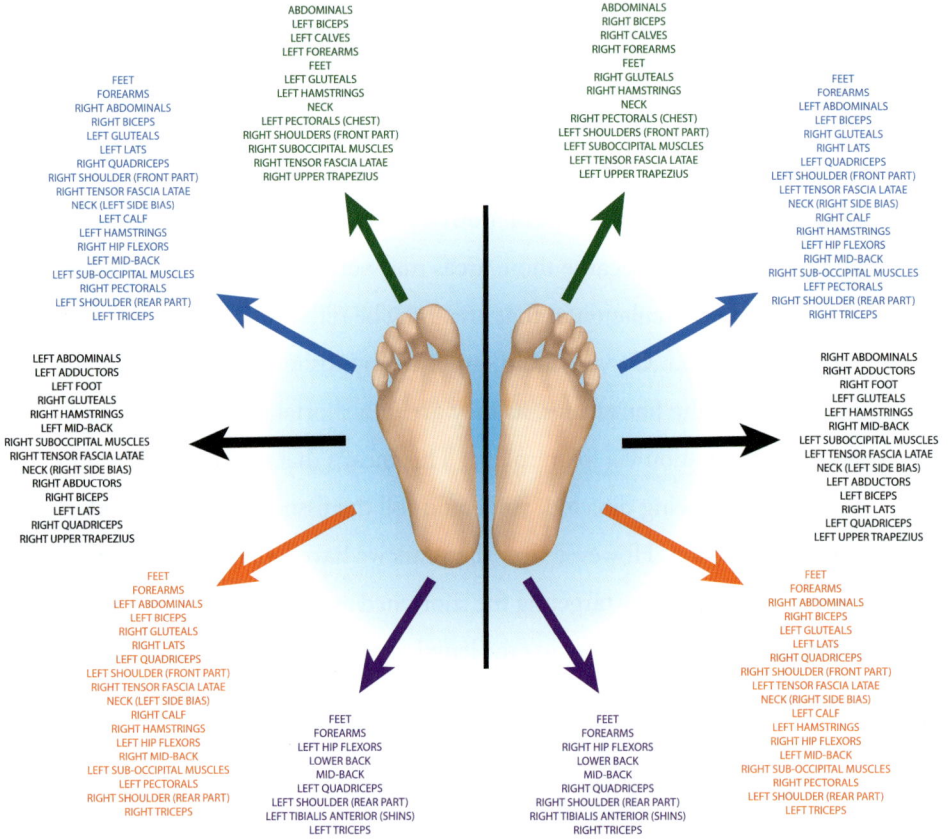

ABDOMINALS
LEFT BICEPS
LEFT CALVES
LEFT FOREARMS
FEET
LEFT GLUTEALS
LEFT HAMSTRINGS
NECK
LEFT PECTORALS (CHEST)
RIGHT SHOULDERS (FRONT PART)
RIGHT SUBOCCIPITAL MUSCLES
RIGHT TENSOR FASCIA LATAE
RIGHT UPPER TRAPEZIUS

ABDOMINALS
RIGHT BICEPS
RIGHT CALVES
RIGHT FOREARMS
FEET
RIGHT GLUTEALS
RIGHT HAMSTRINGS
NECK
RIGHT PECTORALS (CHEST)
LEFT SHOULDERS (FRONT PART)
LEFT SUBOCCIPITAL MUSCLES
LEFT TENSOR FASCIA LATAE
LEFT UPPER TRAPEZIUS

FEET
FOREARMS
RIGHT ABDOMINALS
RIGHT BICEPS
LEFT GLUTEALS
LEFT LATS
RIGHT QUADRICEPS
RIGHT SHOULDER (FRONT PART)
RIGHT TENSOR FASCIA LATAE
NECK (LEFT SIDE BIAS)
LEFT CALF
LEFT HAMSTRINGS
RIGHT HIP FLEXORS
LEFT MID-BACK
LEFT SUB-OCCIPITAL MUSCLES
RIGHT PECTORALS
LEFT SHOULDER (REAR PART)
LEFT TRICEPS

FEET
FOREARMS
LEFT ABDOMINALS
LEFT BICEPS
RIGHT GLUTEALS
RIGHT LATS
LEFT QUADRICEPS
LEFT SHOULDER (FRONT PART)
LEFT TENSOR FASCIA LATAE
NECK (RIGHT SIDE BIAS)
RIGHT CALF
RIGHT HAMSTRINGS
LEFT HIP FLEXORS
RIGHT MID-BACK
RIGHT SUB-OCCIPITAL MUSCLES
LEFT PECTORALS
RIGHT SHOULDER (REAR PART)
RIGHT TRICEPS

LEFT ABDOMINALS
LEFT ADDUCTORS
LEFT FOOT
RIGHT GLUTEALS
RIGHT HAMSTRINGS
LEFT MID-BACK
RIGHT SUBOCCIPITAL MUSCLES
RIGHT TENSOR FASCIA LATAE
NECK (RIGHT SIDE BIAS)
RIGHT ABDUCTORS
RIGHT BICEPS
LEFT LATS
RIGHT QUADRICEPS
RIGHT UPPER TRAPEZIUS

RIGHT ABDOMINALS
RIGHT ADDUCTORS
RIGHT FOOT
LEFT GLUTEALS
LEFT HAMSTRINGS
RIGHT MID-BACK
LEFT SUBOCCIPITAL MUSCLES
LEFT TENSOR FASCIA LATAE
NECK (LEFT SIDE BIAS)
LEFT ABDUCTORS
LEFT BICEPS
RIGHT LATS
LEFT QUADRICEPS
LEFT UPPER TRAPEZIUS

FEET
FOREARMS
LEFT ABDOMINALS
LEFT BICEPS
RIGHT GLUTEALS
RIGHT LATS
LEFT QUADRICEPS
LEFT SHOULDER (FRONT PART)
RIGHT TENSOR FASCIA LATAE
NECK (LEFT SIDE BIAS)
RIGHT CALF
RIGHT HAMSTRINGS
LEFT HIP FLEXORS
RIGHT MID-BACK
LEFT SUB-OCCIPITAL MUSCLES
LEFT PECTORALS
RIGHT SHOULDER (REAR PART)
RIGHT TRICEPS

FEET
FOREARMS
RIGHT ABDOMINALS
RIGHT BICEPS
LEFT GLUTEALS
LEFT LATS
RIGHT QUADRICEPS
RIGHT SHOULDER (FRONT PART)
LEFT TENSOR FASCIA LATAE
NECK (RIGHT SIDE BIAS)
LEFT CALF
LEFT HAMSTRINGS
RIGHT HIP FLEXORS
LEFT MID-BACK
RIGHT SUB-OCCIPITAL MUSCLES
RIGHT PECTORALS
LEFT SHOULDER (REAR PART)
LEFT TRICEPS

FEET
FOREARMS
LEFT HIP FLEXORS
LOWER BACK
MID-BACK
LEFT QUADRICEPS
LEFT SHOULDER (REAR PART)
LEFT TIBIALIS ANTERIOR (SHINS)
LEFT TRICEPS

FEET
FOREARMS
RIGHT HIP FLEXORS
LOWER BACK
MID-BACK
RIGHT QUADRICEPS
RIGHT SHOULDER (REAR PART)
RIGHT TIBIALIS ANTERIOR (SHINS)
RIGHT TRICEPS

FOAM ROLLING TARGETS
LENGTHENED TISSUE
BASED ON FOOT PRESSURES

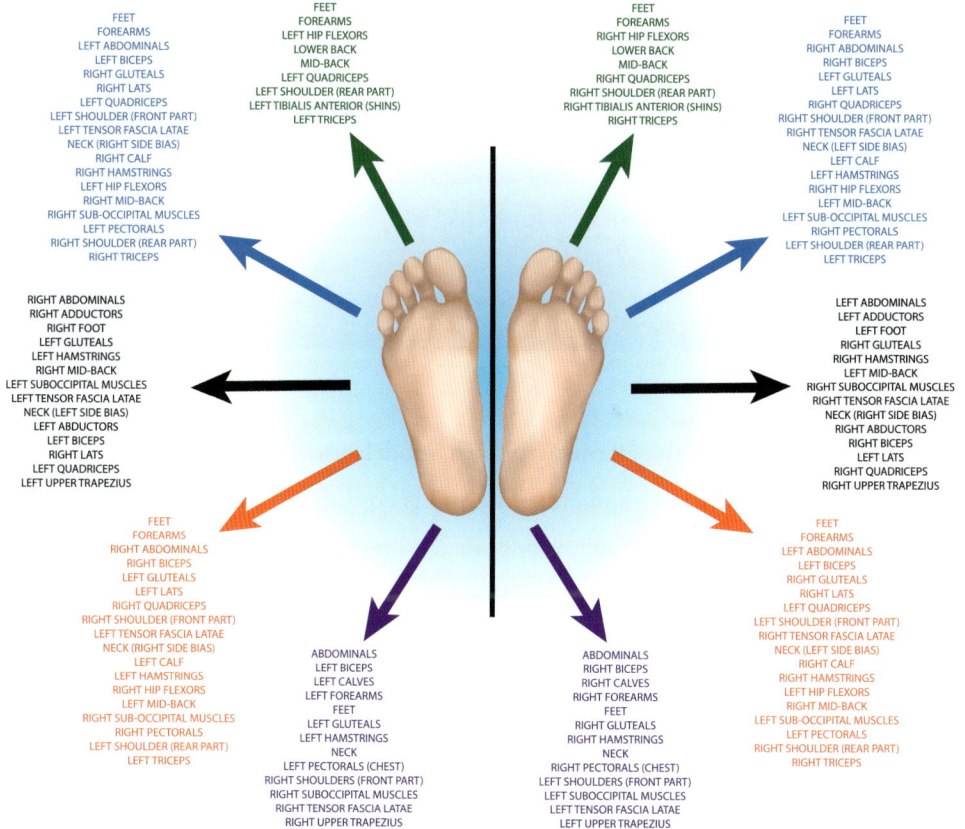

FEET
FOREARMS
LEFT ABDOMINALS
LEFT BICEPS
RIGHT GLUTEALS
RIGHT LATS
LEFT QUADRICEPS
LEFT SHOULDER (FRONT PART)
LEFT TENSOR FASCIA LATAE
NECK (RIGHT SIDE BIAS)
RIGHT CALF
RIGHT HAMSTRINGS
LEFT HIP FLEXORS
RIGHT MID-BACK
RIGHT SUB-OCCIPITAL MUSCLES
LEFT PECTORALS
RIGHT SHOULDER (REAR PART)
RIGHT TRICEPS

FEET
FOREARMS
LEFT HIP FLEXORS
LOWER BACK
MID-BACK
LEFT QUADRICEPS
LEFT SHOULDER (REAR PART)
LEFT TIBIALIS ANTERIOR (SHINS)
LEFT TRICEPS

FEET
FOREARMS
RIGHT HIP FLEXORS
LOWER BACK
MID-BACK
RIGHT QUADRICEPS
RIGHT SHOULDER (REAR PART)
RIGHT TIBIALIS ANTERIOR (SHINS)
RIGHT TRICEPS

FEET
FOREARMS
RIGHT ABDOMINALS
RIGHT BICEPS
LEFT GLUTEALS
LEFT LATS
RIGHT QUADRICEPS
RIGHT SHOULDER (FRONT PART)
RIGHT TENSOR FASCIA LATAE
NECK (LEFT SIDE BIAS)
LEFT CALF
LEFT HAMSTRINGS
RIGHT HIP FLEXORS
LEFT MID-BACK
LEFT SUB-OCCIPITAL MUSCLES
RIGHT PECTORALS
LEFT SHOULDER (REAR PART)
LEFT TRICEPS

RIGHT ABDOMINALS
RIGHT ADDUCTORS
RIGHT FOOT
LEFT GLUTEALS
LEFT HAMSTRINGS
RIGHT MID-BACK
LEFT SUBOCCIPITAL MUSCLES
LEFT TENSOR FASCIA LATAE
NECK (LEFT SIDE BIAS)
LEFT ABDUCTORS
LEFT BICEPS
RIGHT LATS
LEFT QUADRICEPS
LEFT UPPER TRAPEZIUS

LEFT ABDOMINALS
LEFT ADDUCTORS
LEFT FOOT
RIGHT GLUTEALS
RIGHT HAMSTRINGS
LEFT MID-BACK
RIGHT SUBOCCIPITAL MUSCLES
RIGHT TENSOR FASCIA LATAE
NECK (RIGHT SIDE BIAS)
RIGHT ABDUCTORS
RIGHT BICEPS
LEFT LATS
RIGHT QUADRICEPS
RIGHT UPPER TRAPEZIUS

FEET
FOREARMS
RIGHT ABDOMINALS
RIGHT BICEPS
LEFT GLUTEALS
LEFT LATS
RIGHT QUADRICEPS
RIGHT SHOULDER (FRONT PART)
LEFT TENSOR FASCIA LATAE
NECK (RIGHT SIDE BIAS)
LEFT CALF
LEFT HAMSTRINGS
RIGHT HIP FLEXORS
LEFT MID-BACK
RIGHT SUB-OCCIPITAL MUSCLES
RIGHT PECTORALS
LEFT SHOULDER (REAR PART)
LEFT TRICEPS

FEET
FOREARMS
LEFT ABDOMINALS
LEFT BICEPS
RIGHT GLUTEALS
RIGHT LATS
LEFT QUADRICEPS
LEFT SHOULDER (FRONT PART)
RIGHT TENSOR FASCIA LATAE
NECK (LEFT SIDE BIAS)
RIGHT CALF
RIGHT HAMSTRINGS
LEFT HIP FLEXORS
RIGHT MID-BACK
LEFT SUB-OCCIPITAL MUSCLES
LEFT PECTORALS
RIGHT SHOULDER (REAR PART)
RIGHT TRICEPS

ABDOMINALS
LEFT BICEPS
LEFT CALVES
LEFT FOREARMS
FEET
LEFT GLUTEALS
LEFT HAMSTRINGS
LEFT PECTORALS (CHEST)
RIGHT SHOULDERS (FRONT PART)
RIGHT SUBOCCIPITAL MUSCLES
RIGHT TENSOR FASCIA LATAE
RIGHT UPPER TRAPEZIUS

ABDOMINALS
RIGHT BICEPS
RIGHT CALVES
RIGHT FOREARMS
FEET
RIGHT GLUTEALS
RIGHT HAMSTRINGS
NECK
RIGHT PECTORALS (CHEST)
LEFT SHOULDERS (FRONT PART)
LEFT SUBOCCIPITAL MUSCLES
LEFT TENSOR FASCIA LATAE
LEFT UPPER TRAPEZIUS

WHEN FOAM ROLLING, REMEMBER:

- Always check in with where the pressure is in the feet before rolling.
- Determine target areas to roll.
- Go slow enough to feel. Do not roll fast.
- Take your time and use gentle to moderate pressure.
- Do not try and obliterate the sore spots.
- Work around the most tender areas.
- If, over time, you feel the need to apply greater pressure, do so in moderation.
- Be sure to perform a follow-up "check in" to see if the pressure in the feet has changed.
- Observe and be aware of any changes.

In most of the following photos, models use a three-foot foam roll that is six inches in diameter. The roll is considered to have moderate firmness (rolls can be soft, moderate, or hard). There are several other tools that can be used to achieve the same results. In other photos, models use a small inflatable ball or two tennis balls taped together. Following are different methods that can be utilized to enhance soft tissue circulation.

ABDOMINALS

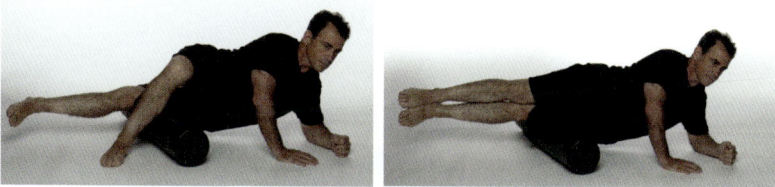

Position the body face down with a small inflatable ball under the belly button. Rest the forehead against the back of both hands. Lower the weight of the body onto the ball. Slowly breathe in and out through the nostrils. Allow the body to sink around the ball with every breath. Repeat several times.

ABDUCTORS

Position the body on one side with the elbow and feet supporting it. Lower the side of the thigh, just below the hip bone (greater trochanter) onto the roll. Slowly roll back and forth along the outer thigh. Repeat several times. For a greater degree of intensity, place the opposite leg on top of the leg that is being rolled.

ADDUCTORS

Place the roll parallel to the body outside of one leg. Bring the leg closest to the roll, up and out away from the body so the inner thigh close to the groin rests on the roll. Support the weight of the body on both hands or

elbows and the opposite leg. Move the body slowly left and right so the inner thigh presses into the roll from the groin to the inside of the knee. Repeat several times.

BICEPS

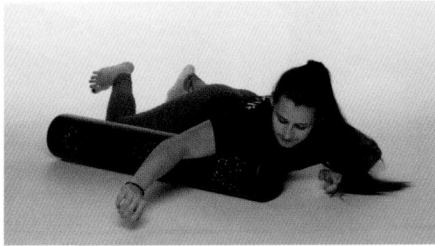

Lie face down with the edge of the roll under the front of the shoulder.

Move the body away from the roll so the pressure travels down the arm to the elbow. The arm can rotate internally or externally to provide greater pressure to the inside or outside of the biceps. Repeat several times.

CALVES

Rest the back of one ankle at the edge of the roll. Support the body with both hands and the opposite leg. Keep the hips off the floor as the hips push away from the hands so the roll moves up the lower leg toward the knee. The leg can rotate inward or outward for greater concentration along the sides of the calf muscles. For greater pressure cross the opposite leg on top of the rolling leg. Repeat several times.

CHEST (PECTORALS)

Lie face down with the edge of the roll under the front of the shoulder. Move the body toward the roll so the pressure travels across the chest to the sternum (breastbone). Repeat several times.

FEET

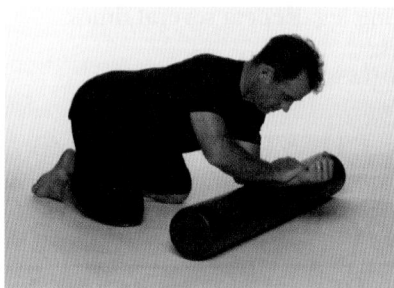

Place a bare foot on a ball or the "peanut" (two tennis balls taped together). Apply bodyweight on the foot as it rolls back and forth from the toe tips to the heel.

FOREARMS

Rest on both knees, with the forearm on the roll. Place the other arm on top of the resting forearm and lean over the roll for greater pressure. Roll the arm back and forth from the wrist to the elbow. Be sure to flip the palm up for several passes and then palm down for several more.

GLUTEALS (MEDIUS AND MAXIMUS)

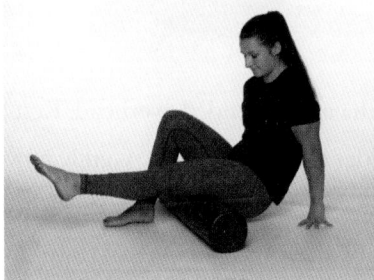

Sit on the roll while leaning back and supporting the upper body with one hand. Rotate the body onto one buttock. For greater intensity the leg of the rolling side can be crossed over the opposite knee. Gently roll back and forth across the entire buttock. The gluteus medius is on the outside portion of the hip and the gluteus maximus is more central and inside. Repeat the rolling action several times.

HAMSTRINGS

Rest the back of one knee at the edge of the roll. Support the body with both hands and the opposite leg. Keep the hips off the floor as the hips push away from the hands so the roll moves up the thigh toward the buttocks. Repeat several times.

HIP FLEXORS

In a quadruped position, lower the crease of the hip at the top of the quadriceps on the corner of roll's end. Support the body on either the hands or elbows. Slowly move the body back and forth from the crease to the belly button and back again. Repeat several times.

LATS

Lie on the side with the arm extended overhead. Rest the armpit and edge of the scapula (shoulder blade) on the roll. Gently move the body back and forth along the underside of the arm and toward the back side of the rib cage. Do not travel too far down into the ribcage because it may be too much pressure and could be injurious to the rib cage. Stop mid-way down the back before changing directions. Next rotate the body upward enough so the pressure travels toward the mid-back region from the pit of the arm. Repeat these actions several times.

MID-BACK
(RHOMBOIDS & LOWER TRAPEZIUS)

In a seated position lay back and rest the top of the lower back against the roll. Support the weight of the head with both hands. Lift the hips off the floor and pull the body toward the feet so the roll travels up the spine. Stop when the roll reaches the top of the neck. The elbows can be out from the body to roll tissue across the scapula. The elbows can also be pulled toward each other to target the tissue between the scapulae.

NECK (CERVICAL SPINE)

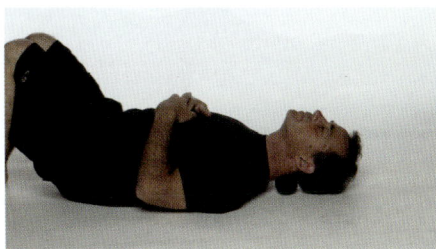

Lie face up with knees bent and feet flat. Place two balls taped together (also called a peanut) under the top portion of the neck. Apply gentle pressure against the balls with the weight of the head. Migrate the body slowly toward the head so the taped balls move down the spine an inch at a time. Repeat these motions several times.

OCCIPUT (BASE OF SKULL)

Lie face up with knees bent and feet flat. Place a small ball, or two balls taped together in a peanut shape, under the top portion of the neck at the base of the skull. Apply gentle pressure against the ball with the weight of the head. Slowly nod the head up and down. Then turn the head left and right. Lastly, side bend the head by pulling one ear toward the shoulder at a time. Repeat these three movements several times.

QUADRICEPS

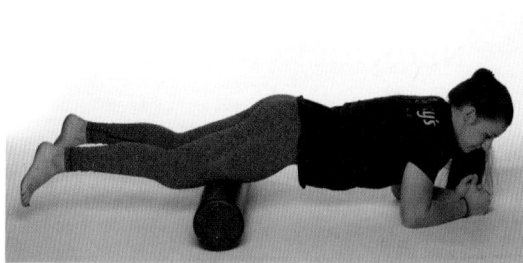

In a quadruped position lower the front of the thigh, just above the patella (knee cap) on the roll. The body can be supported on the hands or elbows. Slowly move the body backward so the roll moves up the thigh. By rotating the leg outward, pressure is applied to the inside portion of the quadriceps. By rotating the leg inward pressure is applied to the outside portion of the quadriceps. For greater overall pressure, the opposite leg can be placed on the rolling leg. Repeat several times.

SHOULDERS (DELTOIDS)

Lie on the side with the arm extended overhead. Rest the armpit and edge of the scapula (shoulder blade) on the roll. Gently move the body back and forth along the underside of the arm. Do *not* travel down into the ribcage because it may be too much pressure and could be injurious to the rib cage. Next rotate the body upward enough so the pressure travels toward the top of the shoulder. Repeat these actions several times.

TFL (TENSOR FASCIA LATAE)

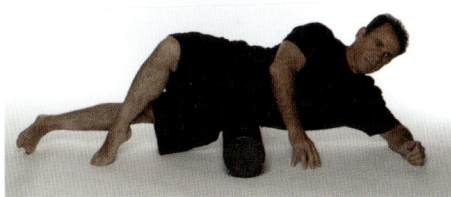

Position the body on one side with the elbow and feet supporting. Lower the side of the hips, between the hip bone and the top of the pelvis, onto the roll. Slowly roll back and forth along the outer hip. Repeat several times.

UPPER TRAPEZIUS

Lie sideways with the side of the head resting on the roll like a pillow. Gently press the neck into the roll as the body travels toward the head and the roll heads toward the shoulder. Repeat several times.

TARGET THE PROBLEM, NOT THE SYMPTOM: ACL TEARS

One of the more common injuries in any sport is tearing the anterior cruciate ligament (ACL). The ACL connects the top front portion of the tibia (shin bone) to the bottom rear part of the femur (thigh bone). Ligaments are tough bands of fibrous tissue that connect bone to bone. Compared to muscles, ligaments stretch very little and do not have as many blood vessels. This means that if too much force is applied to a ligament, it will become sprained, tearing rather than stretching. With few blood vessels in the tissue, the limited circulation means a recovery process that is a lot longer. Usually, surgery is used as a way to reattach torn portions. In some cases where the ACL is unrepairable, surgeons will use ligaments from other areas of the body, or from a cadaver, to create a completely new ACL.

The cause of ACL tears is mainly due to the tibia and femur moving too quickly away from one another. This can happen when both bones rotate in opposite directions. It can also happen when they rotate in the same direction, just at different rates of speed, as when changing directions quickly. Just ask professional athletes like NFL players Julian Edelman or Jimmy Garoppolo, and NBA player Ricky Rubio, who suffered season-ending ACL tears without being contacted by another player. What should ideally control, or decelerate, knee motion are the muscles and fascia which surround the joint. It is similar to the arresting cables that catch jets as they land on an aircraft carrier. This involves tremendous amounts of force that need to slow down real fast. The quadriceps, gluteals, hamstrings, and calf muscles must lengthen in order help decelerate knee flexion and external rotation. If the tissue does not slow down such force, the ligaments will often take the brunt.

Most anatomy books will state the opposite when it comes to knee mechanics and rotation, because the way anatomy is studied is with a cadaver lying on a gurney, not while the body is in motion. These two conditions (lying on a table and moving upright) will bring about two different outcomes and understandings of biomechanics. It is this confusion and incomplete information about movement which still prevails and is the cause of ineffective rehabilitation strategies and conditioning programs to this day. When a body is in motion and the knee flexes and travels medially (toward the midline of the body) the knee joint is externally rotating. As the knee begins to extend (straighten) the joint internally rotates. This is because the femur moves much faster than the tibia.

When a person is standing, and the knee joint is not in its proper structural position, the surrounding muscles will either shorten or lengthen to accommodate the position. Muscles that are too long in a resting state will not have the capacity to properly shorten back to the proper resting length. Muscles that are too short will have difficulty lengthening back to the normal resting length. Neither scenario is ideal. Over time, if this position is reinforced, the length of the muscles becomes normalized, the imbalances are maintained, and the knee resides in a compromised, vulnerable state. The ability to decelerate force wanes. The ACL is just waiting in the shadows ready to snap.

There are several approaches in the fitness and rehab world that claim to help prevent future ACL tears, but most do so by avoiding the movements where bad things can happen. The trouble with this approach is that the neuromuscular system never gets to experience what to do when the knee travels into "foreign territory" and how to decelerate and get out of it. It would be similar to telling a child never to cross a busy intersection. Then, one day a ball bounces out into the intersection and the child, without thinking, charges after it. The potential for major harm is very high. A better approach would be to teach the child how to cross safely so that no matter which street they cross, the chance of success is almost guaranteed. Therefore, we want the knee, and its surrounding tissues, to gain the experience of all types of movement as it relates to the gait cycle. Guide the joint into flexion and rotation and guide it back out again. The nerve endings will feed vital information to the connective tissue to take pressure off the ligaments. This will greatly reduce the likelihood of future non-impact ACL tears.

CHAPTER 5
AUTONOMIC NERVOUS SYSTEM AS A GUIDE

LET YOUR NERVOUS SYSTEM BE YOUR GUIDE

Now that you have gone through the assessments and learned about your posture, foot pressure, and how your body moves (and equally important how it does not), it is time to create your program. The mobility and strength exercises (see Chapters 6 and 7, respectively) can be chosen from the areas where you found the most restrictions or differences. There are two charts for the strength exercises and two for the mobility drills found in the Appendix. The simple answer to the question of "Why are there two charts?" is "If it's not one...it's the other."

- One chart details exercises based on the rule of motion that "joints act and muscles react." In osteopathy, this is considered the "structural approach." The exercises will drive the body into the movements that are missing. The potential result is that the muscles and soft tissue surrounding the moving joints will begin to understand their role in the movement and learn how to properly move again.

- The second chart details exercises based on the rule of motion that states, "Muscles lengthen before they contract." This approach is sometimes called the "functional approach" or Reactive Neuromuscular Training (RNT). The body is driven into the places where it already tends to go. This allows muscles, which may have trouble shortening back to a neutral state, to experience the stretch-shortening reflex, so the muscle learns to contract a little more to return the body back to center.

Which one of the approaches best suits you or area of your body is really up to you. It is not a one-size-fits-all type of thing. For example, while this is not written in stone, the hips and pelvis often react better to the structural approach while the shoulders respond better to the functional approach.

This is why assessing and reassessing movement is important. It will be your guide to determine which movement and which of the two approaches are best suited for your body in that moment. It is possible that you could choose exercises or mobility drills from all four charts. After performing one exercise, reassess the missing movement and feel if the quality of the movement improved. If it improved, great. If it did not, try an exercise from the column of the alternate chart and reassess. No two people have led truly identical lives, even twins. This means every person is unique and how they respond to movement is dependent upon all they have experienced in their life. This means that there is not one program that will work for everyone. It needs to be determined by how your brain and body interpret and respond to what you give it.

Then there is the question of how much weight should be used. How many repetitions are an ideal range? How many sets? What level of intensity? How do you choose? There is no better gauge for determining all of these aspects than the Central Nervous System (CNS). The CNS never sleeps and is constantly regulating strength, mobility, visual acuity, and balance based on the stimuli it receives. The part of the CNS known as the autonomic nervous system (ANS) has evolved automatic and subconscious responses as a means of survival. When the ANS encounters a threat, it creates a sympathetic "fight or flight" response. This helped our ancestors survive injuries, predators, invading armies, extreme weather, and other dangers. There may not be any saber-toothed tigers or invading armies in your daily life, but the ANS response is happening constantly regardless. You might have experienced this "fight or flight" response if you got stopped for a traffic violation, had an argument with your significant other, found an overdue bill notice in the mail, or found yourself walking down a dark alley alone. It also occurs when exercising.

If the ANS detects restricted movement, pain, or structural compromise, it registers as a threat and the "fight or flight" response will be triggered. Your heart rate and blood pressure increase as your breathing shallows (this may be almost imperceptible, but occurs nonetheless). Your muscles tense, your balance diminishes, and your field of vision narrows to focus on the threat that is directly in front of you (having tunnel vision). These are automatic physical responses that occur when your ANS goes into threat mode. The opposite will occur when the ANS senses all is well. Strength will increase. Range of motion will improve. Balance will be better. This response is known as the parasympathetic response. Muscles can tense or relax, balance can improve or become impaired, strength can increase or decrease, and vision can constrict or expand. It all depends on what the autonomic nervous system receives, interprets, and responds to in the moment. The goal is to achieve a balance of sympathetic and parasympathetic responses. A Goldilocks state for the nervous system. Too much of either is not desirable for optimal performance.

This means these responses can be used as a way to test whether or not the exercise you perform is, in that moment in time, considered by the ANS to be beneficial to you or a threat. This also will allow you to dial in the appropriate amount of resistance and volume of work (sets and reps). If too much resistance is used or too many repetitions are performed, the "fight or flight" response will kick in and it will show in the test.

There are several ways to test the ANS, and not every person needs to choose the same test (refer to the "Assessing Nervous System Response" chart later in this chapter). You will need to find one or two tests you prefer and use them as your guide to conditioning. The more often you assess the ANS response, the better you will become at understanding, and predicting, what works for you and what does not. Although it is not essential to perform a test after each set, you may want to begin with testing several times during the workout. This way you will become more familiar with how your body responds. After the first week or two you may prefer to test at the beginning of the workout, halfway through, and at the end of the session. For some who have been using this approach for a long time they are able to intrinsically feel which response is triggered by which exercises. Following are eight tests to choose from and which are compared in the "Assessing Nervous System Response" chart. It is important to choose tests that do not create pain.

> The more often you assess the ANS response, the better you will become at understanding, and predicting, what works for you and what does not.

ASSESSING NERVOUS SYSTEM RESPONSE

BALANCE TEST

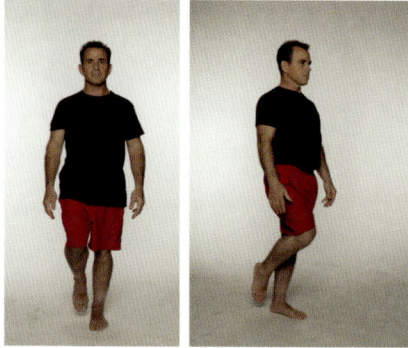

Stand on one leg. How long can you maintain balance? What is the quality of balance like? Is one leg harder to balance upon than the other? This can be your way of assessing the neurological response to exercise. After performing a movement (mobility, strength, or flexibility exercises) repeat the Balance Test, on the more challenged leg, to discern if balance improved or diminished. If it improved, you know that movement was the appropriate selection, duration, and intensity. If it diminished your range of motion, it was either because the exercise itself was not the right

one, or the range of motion, intensity, or duration was too much. You may attempt the same exercise again but try with less range of motion, intensity, or for a shorter period of work.

BODY ROTATION TEST

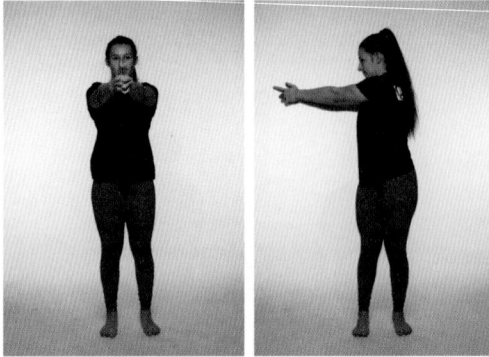

Stand tall with your feet parallel and less than hip width apart. Clasp your hands together with your arms out straight in front of the body at chest level. Gently rotate your body to the left and then to the right. How far can you rotate in each direction? What does the range of motion and level of tension feel like? This can be your way of assessing the neurological response to exercise. After performing a movement (mobility or strength exercises) repeat the Body Rotation Test to discern if the range of motion increased or decreased. If it increased, you know that movement was the appropriate selection, duration, and intensity. If it decreased your range of motion, it was either because the exercise itself was not the right

 one, or the range of motion, intensity, or duration was too much. You may attempt the same exercise again but try with less range of motion, intensity, or for a shorter period of work.

PERIPHERAL VISION TEST

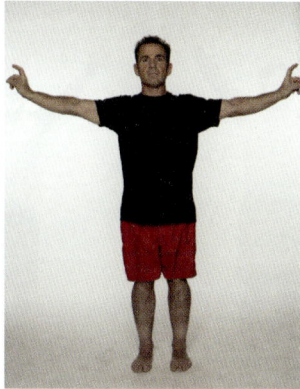

Stand tall with legs straight, feet parallel and less than hip width apart. Keeping the arms straight at the elbows, raise them laterally to shoulder height and back slightly outside your field of vision. Keep the head tall and focus on an object straight ahead across the room. Begin wiggling the fingers as the arms move slowly forward. As soon as you see them in your peripheral vision, stop. How far did the arms move before you saw them? This can be your test. After performing a movement (mobility, strength, or flexibility exercises) repeat the Peripheral Vision Test to discern if the pupils constricted (threat response) or expanded. If peripheral vision expanded, you know that movement was the appropriate selection, duration, and intensity. If it decreased and your arms had to move further forward until they were seen, it was either because the exercise itself was not the right

 one, or the range of motion, intensity, or duration was too much. You may attempt the same exercise again but try with less range of motion, intensity, or for a shorter period of work.

SHOULDER ABDUCTION TEST

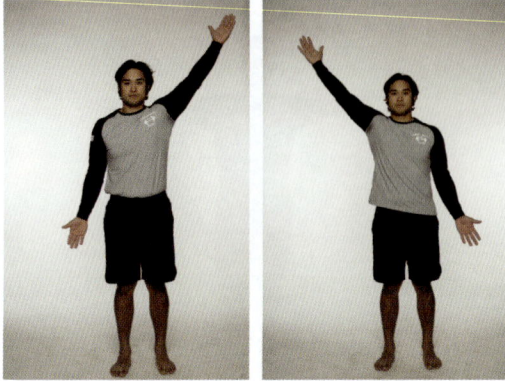

Stand tall with your feet parallel and less than hip width apart. Keeping an arm locked at the elbow, palm facing forward, slowly and gently raise the arm laterally and upward overhead. You can choose one arm or try both. How far can you reach without straining? What does the level of tension feel like? This can be your way of assessing the neurological response to exercise. After performing a movement (mobility or strength exercises) repeat the Shoulder Abduction Test to discern if the range of motion increased or decreased. If it increased, you know that movement was the appropriate selection, duration, and intensity. If it decreased your range of motion, it was either because the exercise itself was not the right

one, or the range of motion, intensity, or duration was too much. You may attempt the same exercise again but try with less range of motion, intensity, or for a shorter period of work.

SHOULDER FLEXION TEST

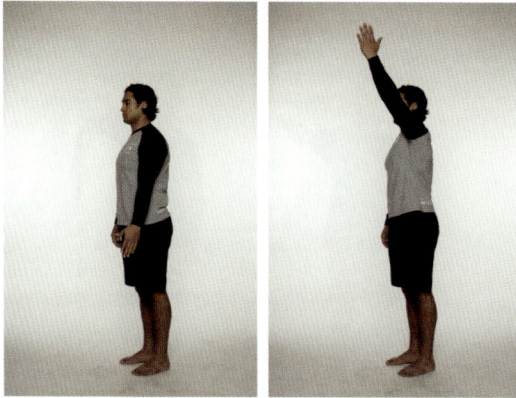

Stand tall with your feet parallel and less than hip width apart. Keeping one arm locked at the elbow, slowly and gently raise the arm forward and upward overhead. You can chose one arm or try both. How far can you reach without straining? What does the level of tension feel like? This can be your way of assessing the neurological response to exercise. After performing a movement (mobility, strength, or flexibility exercises) repeat the Shoulder Flexion Test to discern if the range of motion increased or decreased. If it increased, you know that movement was the appropriate selection, duration, and intensity. If it decreased your range of motion, it was either because the exercise itself was not the right one, or the range

 of motion, intensity, or duration was too much. You may attempt the same exercise again but try with less range of motion, intensity, or for a shorter period of work.

SHOULDER INTERNAL ROTATION (SCARECROW) TEST

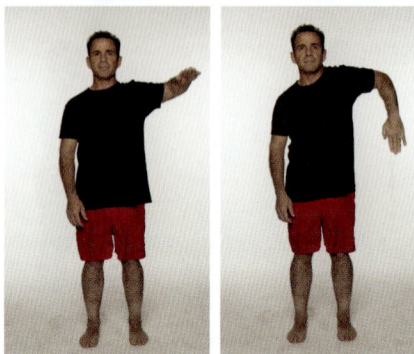

Stand tall with your feet parallel and less than hip width apart. Bring one arm up to shoulder and elbow height. Rotate the arm down but keep the elbow at shoulder height. Do a few repetitions to get a sense of tension. What does the level of tension feel like? How far can you rotate the arm downward without straining? What does the level of tension feel like? Repeat this using the opposite arm. Which arm had the most restriction? This is the arm to use for the test. This can be your way of assessing the neurological response to exercise. After performing a movement (mobility, strength, or flexibility exercises) repeat the Shoulder Internal Rotation Test to discern if the range of motion increased or decreased. If it increased, you know that movement was the appropriate selection, duration, and intensity. If it decreased your range of motion, it was either because the exercise itself was not the right one, or the range of

motion, intensity, or duration was too much. You may attempt the same exercise again but try with less range of motion, intensity, or for a shorter period of work.

STANDING TOE TOUCH TEST

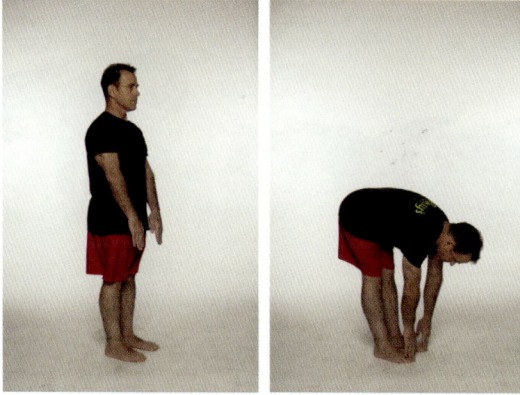

Stand tall with your feet parallel and less than hip width apart. Keep your knees straight as the hips hinge to lower the upper body down. Slowly and gently reach down with both hands toward the toes. Do a few repetitions to get a sense of tension. How far can you reach without bouncing? What does the level of tension feel like? This can be your way of assessing the neurological response to exercise. After performing a movement (mobility or strength exercises) repeat the Standing Toe Touch Test to discern if the range of motion increased or decreased. If it increased, you know that movement was the appropriate selection, duration, and intensity. If it decreased your range of motion, it was either because the exercise itself was not the right one, or the range of motion, intensity, or duration was too much. You may attempt the same exercise again but try with less range of motion, intensity, or for a shorter period of work.

Muscles can tense or relax, balance can improve or become impaired, strength can increase or decrease, and vision can constrict or expand. It all depends on what the autonomic nervous system receives, interprets, and responds to in the moment.

STRENGTH TEST

Choose a strength exercise (such as a push-up, squat, one-arm row, or step-up) that you are able to perform pain free. Perform a certain number of repetitions and gain an experience of the difficulty factor. How hard was it to perform? This can be your test. After performing a movement (mobility, strength, or flexibility exercises) repeat the strength test and discern if it was harder or easier to perform. If it was easier you know that movement was the appropriate selection, duration, and intensity. If the test was harder it was either because the exercise itself was not the right one, or the range of motion, intensity, or duration was too much. You may attempt the same exercise again but try with less range of motion, intensity, or for a shorter period of work. If by altering these elements, the test result improves, then you now know the proper amount of work to apply. If the results do not change, then omit that particular exercise from your program for the time being. Be sure to choose a strength exercise that is not part of your workout. Your results will be thrown off if you performed a set of push-ups and then test with more push-ups.

Assessment	Parasympathetic (What It Wants)	Sympathetic (Threat Response)
BALANCE	Improves	Diminishes
BODY ROTATION	Range of Motion Increases	Range of Motion Decreases
PERIPHERAL VISION	Increase	Decrease
SHOULDER ABDUCTION	Range of Motion Increases	Range of Motion Decreases
SHOULDER FLEXION	Range of Motion Increases	Range of Motion Decreases
SHOULDER INTERNAL ROTATION	Range of Motion Increases	Range of Motion Decreases
STANDING TOE TOUCH	Range of Motion Increases	Range of Motion Decreases
STRENGTH	Strong Response	Weakened Response

TARGET THE PROBLEM, NOT THE SYMPTOM: SPORTS INJURY

A professional athlete I worked with a few years ago had been a national champion of his sport, yet was considering retirement at the age of 30. He had undergone two surgeries to repair the rotator cuff of his right shoulder (the smaller muscles which help maintain the upper arm's position with the collarbone and shoulder blade). The first surgery seemed to be successful at first, but eventually the pain in his shoulder returned. Hence, the need for a second surgery. The same thing happened after the second surgery, and it was suggested he see a different surgeon for a third surgery. Instead, he was encouraged by a friend to pay me a visit.

I asked him about his training routine and exercise selection. In addition to the traditional rubber band therapy exercises he continued to do after his surgeries, he said he did bench press, squats, deadlifts, seated row, biceps curls, triceps pushdowns, lat pulldowns, leg extensions, abdominal crunches, and low back extensions. As you can see, every single exercise was bilateral. Not a single movement trained one arm to swing forward while the other swung back. Not one movement trained the legs to move in opposing directions. Not one movement encouraged the body to rotate. The sport he competed in is performed on a court. His body needed to be able to rotate and move in all three dimensions, not just forward and back. Every single movement in his routine was training his body to minimize rotation and keep his spine still and stable.

We created a timeline of his life with regards to injuries, surgeries, illnesses, etc. We wanted to find out what happened before the shoulder trouble began. The rotator cuff muscles did not just wake up one day and decide to begin giving him trouble. It was probably something that had been going on for quite a while and eventually just reached a breaking point. But what was the underlying reason? The shoulder trouble was a symptom of how his entire body was managing his mass and coordinating his athletic motions. What we discovered was he had broken his big toe on one foot when he was a teenager, long before his shoulder trouble began. His body had to find a new way to move and thus developed a pattern that shifted him off his center to move away from the pain. However, once the pain was gone he kept using the new pattern subconsciously because there was no reason not to. The altered way of moving had normalized and nothing had required any further change. The end result was one of his feet took on more of his weight. One arch began to lift more while the other dropped a little. This change in foot structure encouraged rotation and side-shifting to his entire frame. The pelvis began to rotate in one direction and his rib cage counteracted by rotating in the opposite direction. This, in turn, fed downward back to his feet and encouraged further change. These positions were not dramatic, nor were they noticeable unless you really looked for them. However, even shifting a fraction of an inch off center can have tremendous effects elsewhere. Think of aiming a laser at the center of the moon. If you were to shift the laser just a fraction of a millimeter in your hand the beam will no longer hit the moon. Small changes in one area can have a dramatic effect further along the chain.

His sport required him to be able to rotate evenly left to right, but with the compromised posture that was created, it made that really hard to do, if not impossible. Some muscles had to generate a higher degree of force to overcome the structural distortion. This meant that some were getting overworked while others were being weakened, because they were falling prey to the pulling muscles. Some of the biggest muscles like the gluteals (buttocks) and latissimus dorsi (biggest back muscle) were supposed to slow down his body's mass and momentum during his fast, powerful arm swing. Yet, they were not able to do their job as best they should. This placed a lot more demand on his smaller rotator cuff muscles.

It should be pointed out that after his two surgeries he had gone to physical therapy. There the primary focus was to strengthen his rotator cuff muscles by isolating them with bands and dumbbells. This is often the standard protocol followed and is what is covered by insurance. Many therapists are limited to what they can do with patients based on the person's coverage and what insurance companies allow. At no time did anyone place any value on how the entire body moved in an integrative manner. The only target was the rotator cuff. That would be like putting all of the attention on someone who had just been robbed and not looking for the bandit.

We spent very little time on his shoulder because his shoulder was not the problem. The problem was how his whole body was trying to coordinate movement—beginning with his big toe. Ever since the moment he fractured the big toe, his brain had not wanted to place much pressure in the front portion of that foot. We went through the assessments found in this book, and hunted down the movements he was missing. We created a strength and conditioning routine that addressed the missing components and got him moving more efficiently. Many of the exercises safely guided him on and off the previously injured foot, so the brain realized there was no longer any threat. His shoulder began feeling better immediately. Not a couple of days or a few weeks later…immediately! It has been five years since that first program. He went back on the professional tour within a few months and climbed back up to be in the top five players in the world. He continues to follow these self-guided programs and no longer thinks the worst when physical issues arise. He understands his body is dynamic and in a constant state of change, always orbiting around his center. He understands he has the tools to get his body back to center and perform at the level he requires.

CHAPTER 6
MOBILITY DRILLS

obility is defined as the ability to move freely. As mentioned continuously throughout this book, the human body is at its optimal level for movement, strength, and performance when the joints are in their proper positions and they can move through their ideal range of motion without restriction. In order for proper motion to occur, the muscles that react to joint action must lengthen and shorten without restriction, also.

Newton's third law of motion states that, "For every action there is an equal and opposite reaction." If joint action is restricted, this will demand that one or more other joints increase their range of motion to become hypermobile and move more to compensate. The opposite is also true; when a joint moves too much, another joint will move less. Neither scenario is ideal; that is, a joint that is restricted from its proper action or another joint that reacts more than intended. The body's response in either case is to discover a new way of moving, which inevitably demands more effort and more compensation. This new way of moving, over time, becomes normalized in the brain and is adopted as the assumed movement pattern. Unfortunately, the brain will not correct the compensations on its own. It must be guided back toward center. If left alone, a cycle of compensatory movement patterns will develop other compensations, which will become the "new normal," ultimately leading to degradation, pain, or injury.

Every exercise can also serve as a fantastic assessment, and the ones presented here are no exception. Mobility drills explore how the joints of the body move in relation to each other. Some motions are called "cogs" because most joint motion is similar to cog wheels found in a wrist watch. When one cog wheel moves clockwise the neighboring wheel moves counterclockwise. This can be seen with the pelvis, ribs, and skull when someone is walking with proper gait. These opposing actions occur in all three dimensions of movement.

These mobility drills will enable joints to experience their proper three-dimensional range of motion. The exercises will also enable muscles and other soft tissue to experience a full range of lengthening and shortening in all three dimensions. What often occurs through this series of mobility drills and movement assessments is that the subconscious mind learns to self-correct. It begins to unlock restricted areas of the body. Movement becomes more efficient with less effort. Pain is often reduced or eliminated. Therefore, this should also be considered a valuable part of your overall conditioning program. The more often you assess your movements, the more opportunity the neuromuscular system has to correct inefficient motions, release restricted muscles, and improve coordination.

The two types of mobility drills in this book are known as *open chain* and *closed chain* movements. There can be times when one will benefit the body more than the other.

Open chain drills refer to movements where the segment furthest away from the body, such as the arm or leg, is not connected to the ground or another fixed object. An example would be arm circles or foot circles. The limb is off the floor and the shoulder or ankle is making circular motions. In our regular way of moving, the arms swing freely so many of the mobility drills for the arms and shoulders will be open chain. The legs are more inclined to be closed chain movement because the foot spends more time on the ground than in the air. Many open chain motions tend to isolate one joint at a time. This isolated type of mobility drill is neurologically less demanding and can be considered less intense than many closed chain movements.

Open chain drills can also benefit other joints in the body with which they have a neurological and mechanical relationship. For instance, the left elbow and the right knee have a relationship with one another. This dates back millions of years when we were small mammals roaming on all fours across the primordial forest. The neurological system evolved to bring us upright but the primitive memory still remains. The elbow served as a knee. The wrists and ankles served similar roles, just like the hips and shoulders. In motion, as one elbow bends the opposite knee straightens. Oftentimes, when one joint is encountering movement issues, getting the opposing joint to move can help reduce the issue. So, if the left elbow has trouble extending, a person might try a mobility drill with the right knee and getting it to bend. Then they can reassess the left elbow and see if it made an improvement.

Joint Coupling Relationships

- Wrist & Opposite Ankle
- Elbow & Opposite Knee
- Shoulder & Opposite Hip
- Cervical Spine & S.I. Joint
- Thoracic Spine & Lumbar Spine

Opposing joint relationship

It may seem like magic, but this relationship is firmly based in the science of biomechanics and neurology.

Closed chain movements are when the segment furthest from the body is connected to the ground or fixed object. Closed chain motions involve several joints at one time and are more integrative. Because closed chain movements are not isolating a specific joint, the physical demand for any given muscle is not as much as when working in the open chain motions. They are, however, more demanding neurologically than open chain movements because of the need to coordinate more than one joint.

A natural progression would be to go from open chain to closed chain actions for the lower body and closed to open for the upper body. Ultimately, you will use the assess and reassess process to develop an understanding of which drills are best suited for your body. Do not be surprised if from time to time you need to regress your program rather than make progress. Remember, the body is always adapting to what you experience in life. Sometimes we take two steps forward and one step back. This is a very natural process. There will be times when your progress is slowed or even halted. This is called reaching a plateau. Plateaus may not be desirable but should be expected. It is another way the body is letting you know that it needs a change. The pattern, drill, or exercise needs to be changed.

THE ABILITY OF JOINTS IN THE BODY TO MOVE FREELY MAY BE DICTATED BY AN ASSORTMENT OF THINGS:

- Past or present injuries or trauma
- Joint pain
- Foot pain
- Adaptations to daily environment (e.g., sitting behind a desk or standing in a confined area)
- Fear or emotional insecurity
- Surgical procedures (not limited to joint repair or replacement)
- Inflammation or disease
- Visual or vestibular deficiencies
- Postural distortions
- Neurological disorders
- Malnutrition
- Medications

OPEN CHAIN MOBILITY DRILLS

ANKLE TILTS: Stand tall with feet parallel. In a slow, controlled manner, roll one foot out to the side. The movement is known as inversion and is what typically occurs when a person sprains their ankle. Be sure to place some weight onto the side that is inverting. Return to the starting position.

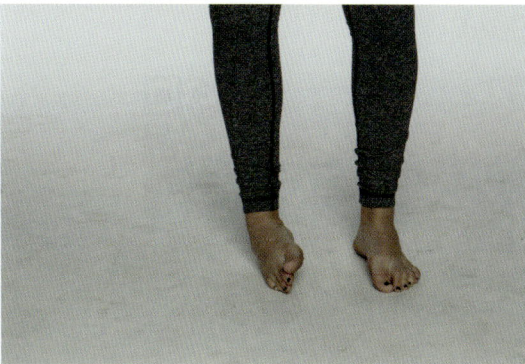

ARM CIRCLES: Stand tall with feet parallel and arms raised out to the sides at shoulder height. With the palms turned down, keep the elbow and wrists rigid and straight. Make small circles forward while maintaining a tall still body. After several circles, flip the palms upward by entirely rotating both arms. Create the same amount of circles backward.

CROSSED KNEE LIFT: Lie on the back with feet flat and knees bent at right angles. Place arms straight out to the sides with palms down. Cross one ankle over the opposite knee. Lift the leg off the floor and bring the knee directly above the same side hip. If the stretch sensation or the muscles around the hip and thigh are too weak, the leg may be supported by placing the foot against a wall or chair. Perform this pose for up to one minute per side. It may be a good idea to perform an additional set on the side that is more restricted.

ELBOW CIRCLES: Raise one arm forward at shoulder height. Make a fist with the raised hand. Bend into the elbow as the fist makes circles as big as possible. Be sure not to move the upper arm or any other part of the body as the circles are performed in both directions.

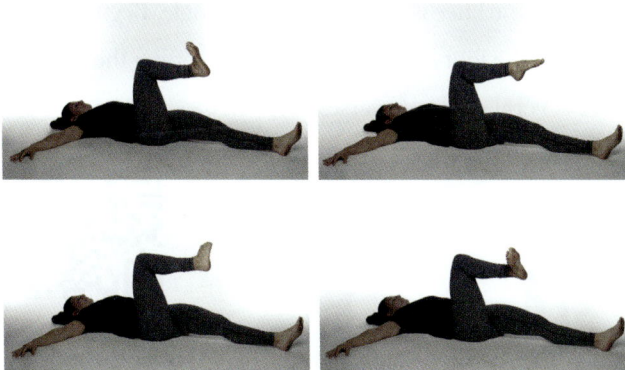

FOOT CIRCLES & FLEXES: Lie face up, with legs extended and resting on the floor. Raise one leg off the floor with the knee bent at a right angle above the hip and foot the same height as the knee. The hip, knee, and ankle should all be forming right angles. Keeping the raised leg as still as possible, begin making slow, perfect circles with the foot. Reverse directions. Next, point and flex the foot north to south.

HIP CIRCLES: Lie face up on the floor with arms out at right angles to the body and knees bents with feet flat. Keep both knees bent and bring them up above the hips. The knees should be directly above the hips with the feet the same height off the floor as the knees. Hips, knees, and ankles should all be at right angles. Slowly bring the knees toward the chest. Separate the legs a few inches and reverse directions until the knees travel past the hips. Bring the legs together and drive them back up toward the chest. After several circles, reverse directions.

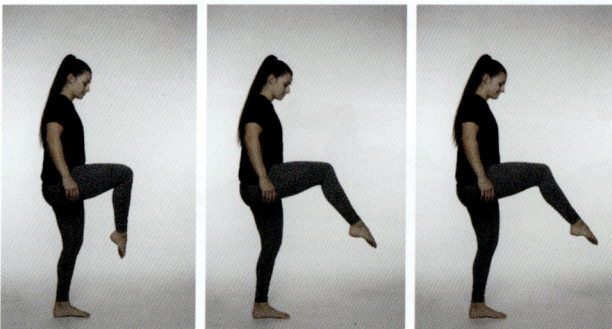

KNEE CIRCLES: Stand tall and relaxed. Lift one leg off the ground and bring the knee up to hip level so the knee is relaxed at a right angle. Begin making large, perfect circles with the foot and lower leg while keeping the thigh as still as possible. After several circles, reverse directions.

NECK GLIDES: Stand tall and relaxed. Glide the head forward and backward without dropping the head or leaning it back. Imagine that a book is resting on the top of the head and should not fall off. Next, glide the head from left to right. Lastly, make circles in both directions.

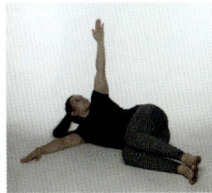

SIDE LYING ARM REACH: Lie on one side of the body in a curled-up position with both knees forward and bent. Rest the head on the bottom arm or a pillow. Reach forward of the body with the top arm touching the floor. Reach upward and over the body to the opposite side. Be sure to create the rotational movement through the rib cage and mid-back more than the arm and shoulder. Return back to the starting position and repeat several times.

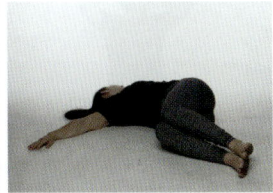

TOE DRAGS: Stand tall and relaxed. Reach back with one leg and the toe pointed straight down. Press down into the floor with the back foot as the body shifts forward. After several repetitions, rotate the back foot outward so the outside of the big toe is contacting the floor. Repeat forward and back shifting motion, dragging the back foot. Next, rotate the back foot inward so the outside of the fifth toe (pinky toe) is contacting the floor. Repeat the same forward and backward motion.

TYPE II SPINE ROTATION: This exercise can be performed seated or standing. Clasp the hands behind the head with elbows out away from the body. In a tall posture, rotate the body in one direction as far as comfortably possible. Perform a gentle side bend and then come up tall. Try and rotate further and perform another side bend. Repeat these actions one more time. Be sure to keep rotating and side bending without returning back to the starting position.

WRIST CIRCLES: Bend at the elbow and bring the wrist up to elbow height to create a right angle at the elbow. With the palm face down, close the hand into a gentle fist. The following motions should occur only at the wrist, with little or no motion at the elbow or shoulder. First, raise the top of the wrist upward. Next, bring the wrist outward. Then drop the wrist downward. Bring the wrist inward and then move it upward to the first position. After several circles, reverse directions.

CLOSED CHAIN MOBILITY DRILLS

ARM WASHRAG: Lie on the back with feet flat and knees bent at right angles. Place the arms out to the side with one hand palm up and one palm down. Slowly begin rotating the arms in opposite directions so the arm with the palm up internally rotates and turns the palm down and vice versa for the other arm. Continue this opposing arm action. Do both arms move identically or is one more restricted? As the arms continue rotating, allow the head to turn toward the palm up side, away from the palm down side. After a few repetitions of head and arm rotations, allow the hips to rotate toward the palm down side (opposite action of the head). Can you experience the washrag-like actions of the arms and spine? Is there any restriction or is there an ease of motion? Perform this action for at least one minute.

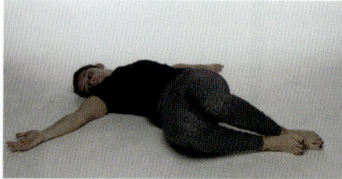

CALVES: Stand facing a wall and take a step back with one leg. Point both feet straight ahead. Maintain a tall posture while slowly and gently moving through the following motions. Perform three to five repetitions of each motion.

FIRST MOTION: Transfer the body's weight over the forward leg. Allow the forward knee to bend while maintaining a straight, extended knee on the rear leg. The heel of the rear foot may lift off the floor slightly.

SECOND MOTION: Keep the weight over the forward foot. Sway the hips from left to right. Reaching overhead with one arm at a time will encourage greater sway if necessary.

THIRD MOTION: Keep the weight over the forward foot. Rotate the pelvis left and right. It might be easier to think about turning the belly button left and right.

CERVICAL SPINE MATRIX: Most neck stretches involve moving the head while the body stays still. Hands are used to pull the head downward or side-to-side. This is fine, but it is missing half of the story. The trouble is when the body is in motion, it is the head which stays still and the body which moves. In everyday movement, the head remains locked on target as the body moves around underneath. These movements will focus on how the neck achieves this ability to keep the head still while moving below.

1ST MOTION: Maintain a level head position at all times, as if a book was balanced on the head. Reach forward with both arms as far as possible. Next, reach back and overhead as far as possible. The rest of the body will need to cooperate by bending forward and back. Be sure to keep the head level and not let the book fall.

2ND MOTION: Maintain a level head position at all times, as if a book was balanced on the head. Cross the arms in front of the chest. Drop one shoulder to the side so the ribs tilt sideways. Reverse directions and tilt the opposite shoulder. Allow the rest of the body to sway below to accommodate the side bending motion.

3RD MOTION: Maintain a level head position at all times, as if a book was balanced on the head. Cross the arms in front of the chest. Rotate the shoulders left and right as far as possible without turning the head. The entire body should rotate left and right except for the head. The head remains static to allow the tissue surrounding the neck and shoulders to experience lengthening and shortening.

CROSSOVER TWIST: Lie on the back with feet flat and knees bent at right angles. Place the arms straight out to the sides with palms down. Cross one ankle over the opposite knee. Rotate the crossed foot and resting leg over to the floor so the leg rests completely to the floor and the foot is flat. Be sure to keep both shoulders on the floor the entire time. If the shoulders are forced to lift off to get the leg and foot to the floor, place a pillow under the rotating leg and foot to keep both shoulders down. Perform this pose for up to one minute per side. It may be a good idea to perform an additional minute on the side that is more restricted.

DOWNWARD DOG: Position the body in a quadruped position on hands and knees. Hands should be placed directly under the shoulders and knees directly under the hips. Hands and knees should be parallel with each other. Slowly press the body back onto the hands and feet, as the knees lift off the floor. The primary focus should be on lengthening the spine and pressing the hips back away from the hands as much as possible. The focus should not be placed on straightening the legs. Often by straightening the legs the back will lose its posture and the pose will be compromised. It is acceptable to maintain a soft bend to both knees provided the spine is lengthening. Maintain this pose for up to one minute.

ELBOW TOUCHES: Stand against a wall with the hips, shoulders, and back of the head in contact with the wall. If possible, have the heels also against the wall unless it causes the other body parts to pull away. Curl the fingers in and place the first two knuckles against the temples with the palms facing forward. Bring both elbows forward until they contact each other. The knuckles should act as hinges and not pull away from the temples at any point in time. Bring the elbows back to the wall. Perform several repetitions. Additional sets may be added for higher level of demand.

FLOOR COGS: Lie on the back with feet flat and knees bent at right angles. You can place the arms gently by the side, with hands resting on the mid-section, or out away from the body at right angles. Slowly tilt the pelvis forward toward the feet so the lower back begins to lift off the floor. Move the pelvis in the opposite direction and feel the lower back return back to the floor. Can you experience the rib cage lift and lower at the same time as the pelvis? Can you experience the head and pelvis move in the same direction at the same time? Perform this movement for at least one minute.

FRONTAL ARM COGS: Stand with feet pointing straight ahead and legs parallel. Keep the head level as if a book was balanced on the crown. Imagine that you are standing in a narrow hallway where there is only room for lateral motion of the body. Raise both arms out to the side at shoulder height with one palm rotated externally upward while the opposite arm is raised with the palm rotated internally downward. Begin rotating the arms in opposing directions. Feel how the motion of the arms drives movement through the rest of the body all the way down to the feet. Try and create as much distance between the hands as possible. Perform several of these arm actions. After, check in with the pressure in your feet and your posture. Has anything changed?

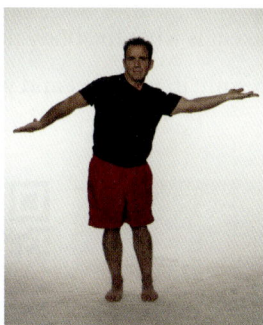

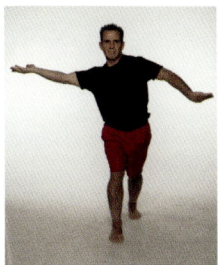

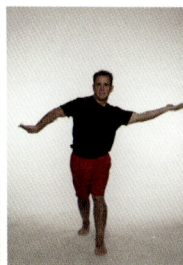

FRONTAL ARM COGS, SPLIT STANCE VARIATION: Perform the same movements with the legs in a forward split stance. Be sure to switch legs to experience the difference and to determine if one stance is more beneficial than the other. Perform several of these arm actions. After, check in with the pressure in your feet and your posture. Has anything changed?

FRONTAL COGS HIKE/DROP: Stand with feet pointing straight ahead and legs parallel. Keep the head level as if a book was balanced on the crown. Imagine that you are standing in a very narrow hallway where there is only room to move sideways without any rotation. Slowly bend one knee and experience the hip drop. As the hip drops, do you get the sense of the pelvis tilting sideways? Simultaneously tilt the ribs in the opposite direction. Be sure to keep the head level as the ribs tilt. Perform the same action on the opposite side. Are both sides equal or does the body easily fall off to one side while requiring a little more effort in the opposite direction? To help encourage this motion, the arm on the side of the bending knee can be raised high overhead. Is there a different experience between each arm raise? Does one side feel like it is what the body needs more than the other? After, check in with the pressure in your feet and your posture. Has anything changed?

FRONTAL COGS VARIATION: Perform the same movements with the legs in a forward split stance. Be sure to switch legs to experience the difference. After, check in with the pressure in your feet and your posture. Has anything changed?

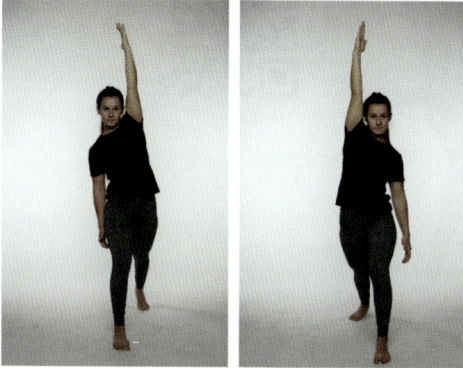

FRONTAL COGS SWAY: Stand with feet pointing straight ahead and legs parallel. Keep the head level as if a book was balanced on the crown. Imagine that you are standing in a very narrow hallway where there is only room to move sideways without any forward or backward action nor any rotation. Slowly shift the pelvis off to one side and then to the other. How do the side motions compare? Does the body easily fall off to one side while requiring a little effort in the opposite direction? Where is the pressure in the feet as the hips travel side to side? Can you keep equal pressure in both feet throughout the whole movement?

As the hips travel to the left, can you experience the ribs tilting in the opposite direction? To further encourage this reaction, you may use the arm to reach. Therefore, if the hips travel left the right arm may reach out to the right. Did this help? Are you able to do this motion evenly in both directions or is there a difference? Does the head stay level in each direction or does it tilt? When the hips travel left does the head travel right and line up directly over the right foot? Does the same occur in the opposite direction? Does one side feel like it is what the body needs more than the other? After, check in with the pressure in your feet and your posture. Has anything changed?

FRONTAL COGS VARIATION: Perform the same movements with the legs in a forward split stance. Be sure to switch legs to experience the difference. After, check in with the pressure in your feet and your posture. Has anything changed?

GLUTEALS: Stand tall with feet parallel. Slide one foot back behind the body and slightly across to the opposite side as far as possible (this movement may be better executed with the sliding foot resting on a plastic furniture mover or a wax paper plate). Reach forward with the same-side arm as the back foot, with the palm turned upward. Attempt to create as much distance between the reaching hand and the sliding foot. Allow the torso to turn in the direction of the forward leg.

HAMSTRINGS MATRIX: Stand on one leg with the opposite leg resting on a chair or box. The raised leg needs to maintain a straight, extended knee position at all times. The standing leg can be softly bent at the knee so the muscles support the weight of the body. For added support, it is best to perform this in a place where one hand can hold on to an immovable object, such as a door frame or countertop. While maintaining this position, perform the following three movements:

FIRST REACHING MOTION: Reach forward in an alternating fashion with one arm at a time. The goal is not to reach as far as possible and create a burning or tearing sort of stretch. The goal is to gain an experience of how the hamstring muscles lengthen while bearing a bit of the body's weight. The sensation should not be painful, but inviting. If it is not inviting the likelihood of the muscles shortening, rather than lengthening, is greater, and is counterproductive to the goal. Breathe out as the arm reaches forward and inhale on the return. Perform three to five repetitions with each arm.

SECOND REACHING MOTION: Reach up and overhead toward the opposite side with one arm. Allow the body to side bend in the direction of the reach while the hips travel away from the reach. Switch arms and reach in the opposite direction. One side will most likely be easier to move toward as the hips will be able to travel further to the side of the elevated leg. Maintain a purely sideways motion with no rotation. Perform three to five repetitions with each arm.

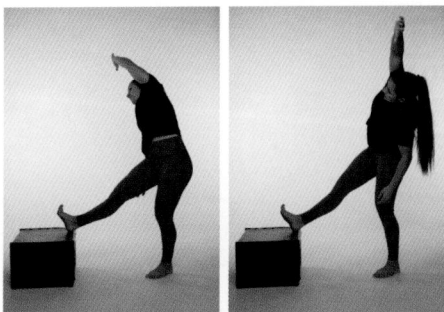

THIRD REACHING MOTION: Reach one hand across the body to create a rotational motion. Allow the pelvis to rotate with the movement. The ribs should rotate more than the hips. Be sure to keep a tall posture during the reaching action. Perform three to five repetitions with each arm.

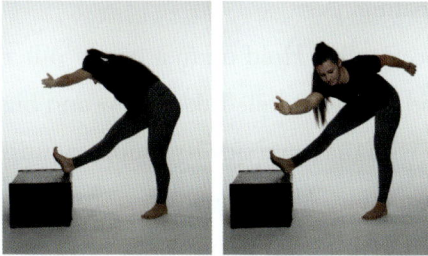

LATS: The following movements may be performed without support after some time, yet when beginning, it is preferred to have something to hold on to. Slowly and gently move through the following motions. Perform three to five repetitions of each motion.

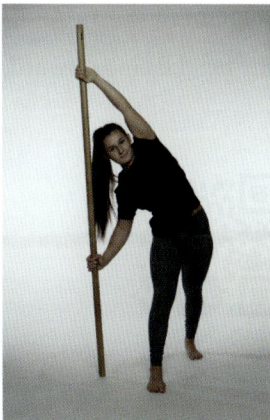

FIRST MOTION: Stand in a split stance under the threshold of a door with both feet pointing straight ahead and the back leg straight at the knee. The heel of the rear foot may lift off the floor slightly. Reach overhead and grip on to the door frame with the arm of the back leg side. The opposite arm should be braced against the frame also. With the help of the bracing arm, press the hips away and then return. Do your best to prevent the body from rotating, making a purely sideways action. Return to the starting position before repeating.

SECOND MOTION: Stand tall with feet parallel. Hold on to a bar or other static, secure object with one hand at waist level. Take a slow and big step back and to the opposite side with the same side leg. Support most of the body's weight on the opposite leg. Allow the torso to rotate in the direction of the holding arm as the distance between the hand and foot becomes as great as possible. Return to the starting position before repeating.

PECTORALS (CHEST): Stand in a forward split stance with the same-side arm of the forward leg raised at shoulder height. Flip the palm upward and feel the chest rise gently. Slowly glide the body forward over the front foot as the arm sweeps backward behind the body. Allow the rib cage to rotate along with the arm. Keep the head facing forward. Return to the starting position and repeat.

QUADRICEPS: Lower the body on to one knee with the opposite leg forward and foot flat. It may be more comfortable to rest the knee on a pillow or cushion. Maintain a tall posture while slowly and gently moving through the following motions. Perform three to five repetitions of each motion.

FIRST MOTION: Glide the pelvis forward and back. Do not allow the pelvis to tilt forward but keep it level.

SECOND MOTION: Sway the hips from left to right. Reaching overhead with one arm at a time will encourage greater sway if necessary.

THIRD MOTION: Rotate the pelvis left and right. It might be easier to think about turning the belly button left and right.

QUAD COGS (A.K.A. CATS & DOGS): Position the body in a quadruped position on hands and knees. Hands should be placed directly under the shoulders and knees directly under the hips. Hands and knees should be parallel with each other. Exhale as the spine lifts upward as evenly as possible. The spine should resemble a half circle and not be flat in any area. Inhale as the spine reverses direction and lowers into the opposite position. At the bottom of the motion the spine should also resemble a half circle (in the opposite direction) and not be flat in any area.

SAGITTAL ARM COGS: Stand with feet pointing straight ahead and legs parallel. Keep the head level as if a book was balanced on the crown. With the arms hanging by your sides, rotate the arms internally as far as possible. Feel how the motion drives the shoulders forward and upward. This causes the ribs to tilt forward and downward and flexes the spine. This in turn causes the pelvis to posteriorly tilt (tucking the tailbone down) and the knees to straighten. Return to the starting position and begin to externally rotate the arms as far as possible. Feel how the motion drives the shoulders backward and down so the shoulder blades pinch together. This causes the ribs to tilt backward and lifts the chest and extends the spine. This in turn causes the pelvis to anteriorly tilt (belly sticks out) and the knees to bend. Perform several of these arm actions. After, check in with the pressure in your feet and your posture. Has anything changed?

SAGITTAL ARM COGS VARIATION: Perform the same movements with the legs in a forward split stance. Be sure to switch legs to experience the difference. Perform several of these arm actions. After, check in with the pressure in your feet and your posture. Has anything changed?

SAGITTAL ARM COGS IN OPPOSITION: Stand with feet pointing straight ahead and legs parallel. Raise one arm forward to shoulder height with the palm rotating externally upward while the opposite arm slowly swings backward with the palm rotating internally downward. The elbow of the forward arm begins to flex as the back arm begins to extend. Try and create as much distance between the hands as possible. Keeping the head still and facing forward, can you experience how the rib cage and spine begin to rotate? Feel how the arm motions drive movement through the rest of the body all the way down to the feet. Once the arms reach their end range of motion, begin to reverse directions so the back arm raises forward and the forward arm travels back. Be sure to explore the end range of movement in each direction and be aware of any differences between sides. After, check in with the pressure in your feet and your posture. Has anything changed?

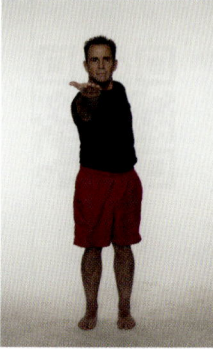

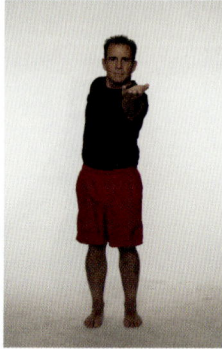

SAGITTAL ARM COGS IN OPPOSITION VARIATION: Perform the same movements with the legs in a forward split stance. Be sure to switch legs to experience the difference. Perform several of these arm actions. After, check in with the pressure in your feet and your posture. Has anything changed?

SAGITTAL COGS: Stand with feet pointing straight ahead and legs parallel. Keep the head still as if a book was balanced on the crown. Slowly tilt the pelvis forward (as if it were a bowl of milk and the milk would pour out of the belly button). Reverse directions and tilt the pelvis backward (so the milk would pour out the tailbone). Do not attempt to go as far as possible. Instead, gain a better understanding of how the pelvis moves in both directions. Is one direction smooth and fluid while the other direction requires more effort to accomplish? Is there pain in one direction? Remember **NOT** to travel into the pain; stop before it is felt! What adjectives would you choose to describe this forward and back action? What is the quality of motion like?

Now bring attention to the ribs as the pelvis continues to gently tilt forward and back. Can you experience your ribs and chest lifting as the pelvis tilts forward (milk out the belly button)? Do you experience the ribs and chest lowering as the pelvis moves in the opposite direction? What is the quality of rib motion like? Does it cause the back muscles to jam up? Does it cause a stretch to be felt? Are the ribs able to keep their position above the pelvis or does it bow forward or lean back when it moves? Do you gain the experience that the ribs and pelvis move in opposition with each other? Does this action feel natural or foreign?

Now bring your attention to your head. Are you able to keep the pelvis tilting and the ribs moving in opposition while keeping the head still and balanced? Do the ribs lift toward the chin when the pelvis tilts forward? Does the chest drop away from the chin when the pelvis tilts back? How would you describe the forward motion compared to the backward motion?

In normal human motion the skull and pelvis move in the same direction while the ribs oppose the action. Is this occurring in your body or is there restriction? Does it require conscious effort or is it natural and fluid? Does one direction feel like it is what the body needs more than the other? After, check in with the pressure in your feet and your posture. Has anything changed?

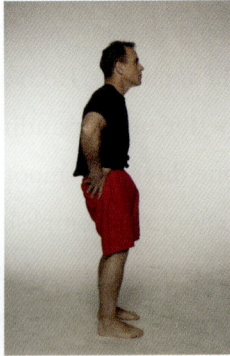

SAGITTAL COGS VARIATION: Perform the identical actions in a split stance with one foot forward of the other (as if you simply took a step forward with

your leg). Next, switch lead legs and try the motions once more. Is there a difference between each side? After, check in with the pressure in your feet and your posture. Has anything changed?

SEATED HIP MOBILITY: Sit tall with knees bent pointing in the same direction. The sole of one foot should be in contact with the knee and thigh of the opposite leg. Lift both knees off the floor and rotate them up and over to the opposite side, so the legs finish in the same position in the opposite direction. Hands may support the body as the legs rotate back and forth. For a higher level of demand, do not use hands for support. Perform this motion for one minute.

SHIFT: Stand in a forward split stance with feet slightly wider than average. Reach upward with the same-side arm of the forward leg. Can you feel that by reaching upward this causes the ribs to tilt laterally to the opposite side? Begin slowly gliding your body forward toward the front foot. Allow the knee to bend forward in the direction of the big toe. Keep the back knee straight but allow the heel to lift off the floor as the body moves forward. Do not allow the pad behind your small toe (5th metatarsal head) to lose contact with the ground. Can you experience the pelvis gliding forward and staying level without tilting to the side? Once these elements are established, raise the lower arm forward with the arm externally rotated and the palm facing upward. As the body glides forward, reach forward and as the body glides back, allow the arm to lower back down.

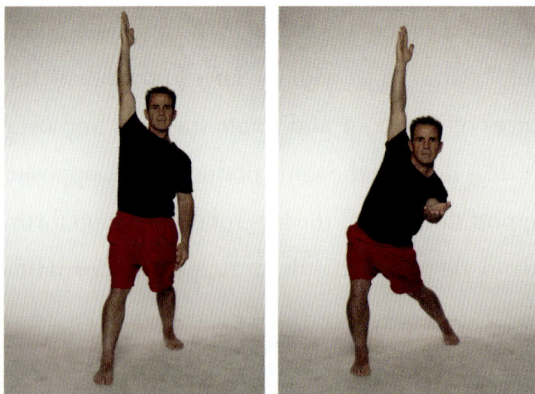

TRANSVERSE ARM COGS: Stand with feet pointing straight ahead and legs parallel. Keep the head level as if a book was balanced on the crown. Imagine that you are standing in a vertical tube where there is only room for rotation of the body, but the arms may reach outside of the tube. Raise one arm forward to shoulder height with the palm rotating externally upward. Reach back around the body with the extended arm. Feel how the arm motions drive movement through the rest of the body all the way down to the feet. Can you experience the spine extending? Return to the starting position and internally rotate the arm so the palm is face down. Reach across the body and around to the opposite side. Can you experience the spine flexing? Be sure to keep tall through the body, allowing only for rotation as the arms reach. Perform several of these arm actions. After, check in with the pressure in your feet and your posture. Has anything changed?

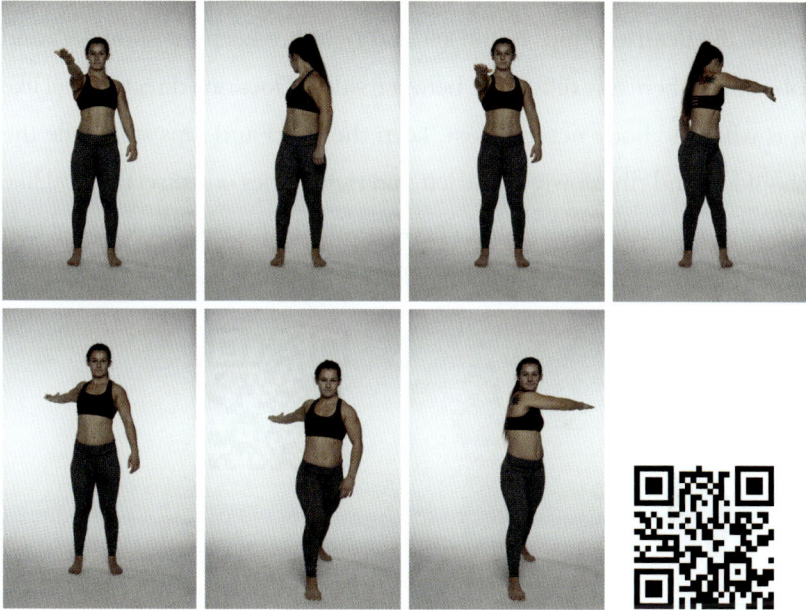

TRANSVERSE ARM COGS VARIATION: Perform the same movements with the legs in a forward split stance. Be sure to switch legs to experience the difference. Perform several of these arm actions. After, check in with the pressure in your feet and your posture. Has anything changed?

TRANSVERSE COGS: Stand with feet pointing straight ahead and legs parallel. Keep the head level as if a book was balanced on the crown. Imagine that you are standing in a vertical tube or phone booth where there is only room for rotation without bending or leaning off the central axis. Slowly rotate the head and hips to the left and right but keep the shoulders and ribs still. Is there any difference between sides? Does one direction feel like it is what the body needs? Next, keep the head and hips still while the shoulders and ribs slowly rotate left and right. Does one direction feel like it is what the body needs? After, check in with the pressure in your feet and your posture. Has anything changed?

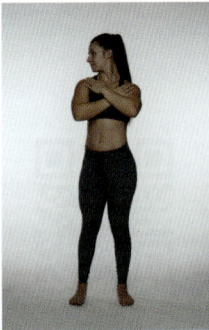

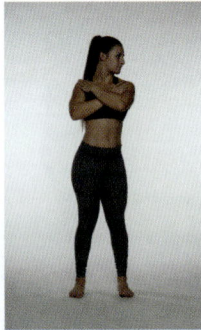

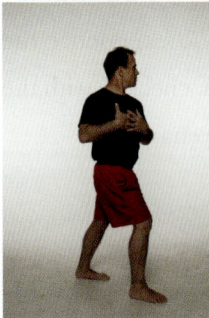

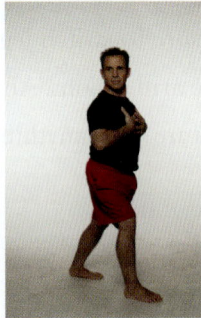

TRANSVERSE COGS VARIATION: Perform the same movements with the legs in a forward split stance. Be sure to switch legs to experience the difference. After, check in with the pressure in your feet and your posture. Has anything changed?

T-SPINE MOBILITY IN QUADRUPED: Position the body in a quadruped position on hands and knees. Hands should be placed directly under the shoulders and knees directly under the hips. Hands and knees should be parallel with each other. Lift one hand off the floor and place it either behind the neck or lower back. Press through the floor with the other arm as the torso and ribs rotate up and away from the floor. Return back to the starting position. Perform five to ten repetitions.

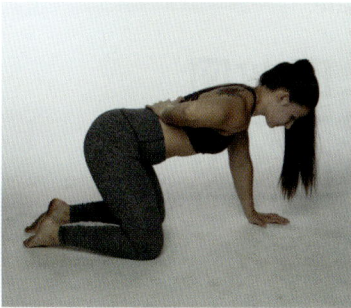

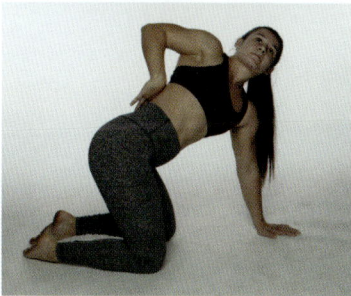

WALL COGS: Stand against a wall with the hips, shoulders, and back of the head in contact with the wall. Keep the heels a few inches off the wall so it does not cause the other body parts to press off the wall. Nod the head forward so the chin drops toward the chest. Next, lift the head in the opposite direction and feel the back of the head slide down the wall. Can you experience the rib cage lift and lower as the head nods up and down? Can you experience the spine moving away and toward the wall? Perform this motion for at least one minute.

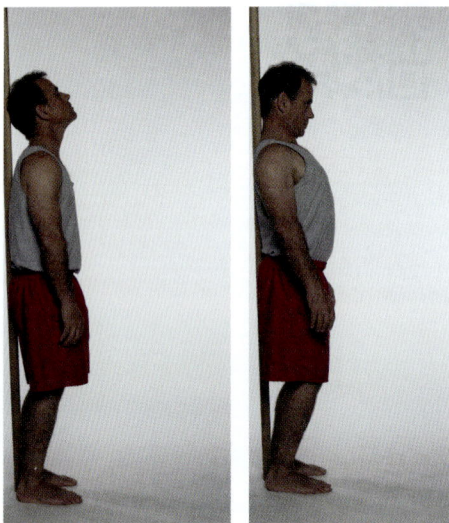

TARGET THE PROBLEM, NOT THE SYMPTOM: THE HEAD LOCKS ON THE HORIZON

I was coaching my son's competitive soccer team several years back. The boys on the team were all eight and nine years old. While the other coach was having the team perform practice drills, one of the fathers on the team came up to me. He told me that his son had just come from the doctor's office. He had been complaining of a pain in his neck. He had been diagnosed with a pinched nerve.

They determined that how this happened was because he sat in his classroom all day turning his head left to pay attention to his teacher. The teacher hadn't considered the potential ramifications of organizing the desks in a horseshoe-shaped layout. The purpose of the arrangement was so students could face one another for optimal class participation. Unfortunately, the room layout caused a majority of students to twist their head in one direction when the teacher gave lessons at the front of the room. The result for at least one student was to develop a really stiff neck.

I asked the father if the doctor had given our young soccer star any exercises to relieve the issue. He replied yes, and demonstrated a couple of the stretches. The dad began by taking one hand and grabbing the side of his head and pulling it down to one side or the other. Then he grabbed the back of his head and began pulling his chin to his chest. He asked me what I thought of the exercises as my face twisted. Here is what I told him.

"Although the head can be a bobblehead and tilt forward and backward, side bend to the left and right, and turn side to side, that isn't how movement primarily occurs for the head and body. If you watch your son out on the field right now, what do you see? Is his head moving in all of those directions or is it staying pretty still while his body does all of the moving? His eyes stay fixed on his target and so does his head. Now, as his target moves his head will follow, but his body will come around to face the target, too.

"It's not that the stretches the doctor gave your son are bad, it is that they do not take into consideration how the body actually moves. They are just based on what his old medical school anatomy books told him. The trouble with most anatomy books is that they base most of the information on studying cadavers on an examination table and not living human bodies as they are in motion. Therefore, how muscles are explained in the anatomy books are just partially correct and incomplete. The muscles of the neck will pull the head in all the directions, like the doctor encouraged. However, more often, the way the muscles work is to keep the head locked on the horizon while the body moves in many directions below it."

I asked the father if he would be okay if I gave his son a few movements to help unlock his neck to "un-pinch" the nerve. With his approval, here's what we did. I grabbed one of the practice cones off the field and placed it on the top of the boy's head. I said, "We're going to play a little game now. Don't let the cone fall off your head." I asked him to bow forward. On his first attempt the cone fell off. By the second attempt he figured out that he had to keep his head level at all times in order for the cone to stay on his head. Next, I asked him to bend back like he was in a limbo contest and then come back up. We did these actions several times without any pain. Then I asked him to lean his body sideways to the left and right. The cone fell off his head again and again until he figured out what he had to do to keep it there. He performed these actions several times without pain. Finally, I asked him to keep his head forward and reach his left arm across to his right and then right arm across to his left and then reach his left arm back around to the left and the same movement with his right arm reaching back and right. His whole body was pivoting underneath a level head. We checked in to see how things felt and a smile began to appear on his face. No more pinching pain. I encouraged him to keep doing this fun game and try a different object next time that was a little harder to balance.

What we really did was reeducate his nervous system and his supporting tissue to perform its primary purpose of maintaining a level head while the body is in motion. When the body is reminded of how it should move with the least restriction, it tends to want to do it more. It was cool that we could make a game out of it so it was not just some boring exercises an adult told him he had to do.

CHAPTER 7
STRENGTH TRAINING

The purpose of strength training should be to encourage the entire body to have stronger, more controlled, and efficient movement with the least amount of restriction and wasted energy. The current approach found in most gyms often falls short of achieving this purpose. Many training programs unknowingly reinforce muscular imbalances, even though the body does grow stronger because of the training. The resulting effect of the common approach will be a body that is structurally compromised and that trains under greater and greater loads. Eventually, the strain will become too much and something is going to crumble.

The exercises in this chapter are all about training the body to transfer force from the nose to the toes and back again with the most efficiency possible. It is also about experiencing the journey the body takes away from center and the journey it takes to return. This means that the strength training exercises may not be traditional lifts like barbell curls, bench press, or lateral raises. This is not to say that such exercises are a waste of time, but you will not find many in these pages. There are plenty of books that can explain all about the nuances of the bench press, seated row, and overhead squat. Let's be clear, there is no such thing as a bad exercise! It all depends on the body that is performing the exercise. Not every exercise will be beneficial for everyone at a given time. However, as the body adapts to this new method of training, it is not out of the question for some exercises, which once brought on pain, to no longer do so.

All the exercises in this chapter have a couple of things in common: they are all derived from the pillars of human movement and they are all components of the gait cycle. The pillars are the basic fundamental movements all humans should be able to perform: moving up and down (often referred to as level changes), pressing or pushing, pulling, and rotation. The other pillar of movement is locomotion, that is, moving the body through space. Whereas most of the exercises here do encourage moving through space, that category is folded into the other four pillars. Gait mechanics are a critical piece in this approach to strength training. If you are unable to perform proper gait patterns, how can you expect to run, play, or do just about anything else? The strength moves will encourage and explore elements of gait motion and progressively combine them together. The moves will connect pieces of the puzzle so you see the entire picture.

Included here also are traditional bilateral actions that most gym goers are used to. While these bilateral actions have an important place in strength programs, they should not be the sole bedrock of anyone's program. It might be better to consider the bilateral exercises as complementary lifts as the body returns closer to center. They should make up about 20 percent to 25 percent of a strength program at the most. Unilateral (one side) and contralateral (opposing sides) exercises are the chief focus for almost every program. Also, it is the *movement* that is also the focus rather than the *muscle*. Many of the exercises provided here will break away from the old-fashioned, linear direction of forward and back. Some will explore strength levels when the body moves laterally, while others will encourage strength during rotation. Several other movements will encourage strength during a combination of all three dimensions at the same time.

Since you may not be familiar with some of the movements here and which require a good deal of coordination, you might find that just using your body weight (without any dumbbells or bands) will be a sufficient level of resistance. This is why most of the photographs have the model performing the movement without dumbbells. The goal with this program is multifaceted: to improve structural integrity, to reduce compensatory patterns, to unlock restricted motions, to allow the force produced by the body to flow with minimal loss of energy, to enhance a balance of tension in the muscular system, and in so doing, ultimately improve full body neuromuscular strength and endurance.

UPPER BODY ACTIONS

Most traditional lifts encourage the body to become rigid during a heavy lift. By remaining rigid, the body gets trained to brace for protection. Rigid bracing is essential for Strongman competitions, but the body may move much differently with activities of daily life or sports. How often during a sport or daily activity would someone find themselves needing to brace in a standing posture like a weightlifter? Let us break away from that approach. It has its place, but it is only one side of the coin. Bracing for impact is great practice but can you be strong without bracing? Are you able to achieve three-dimensional dynamic strength? If you were a boxer, bracing would help you take a punch. But would you want to stay still and brace when you throw a punch? No, you would want the force of your entire body to combine to deliver the knockout blow. You would want the arm to drive forward as the torso rotates, the hips drive upward, and the legs extend so that you connect all the segments of the body to generate force. Just try punching a bag while keeping the rest of the body still.

When an arm exerts force *away* from center it is known as *pressing*. When it exerts force *toward* center it is known as *pulling*. It is ideal to have a balance between pressing and pulling. As the arm moves through space it can dictate how other areas move, creating chain reactions throughout the entire body. This means the arm action can promote missing movements elsewhere. When the arm reaches to the side or overhead it will encourage the torso to move in the direction the arm travels. Meanwhile, the pelvis will travel in the opposite direction to help maintain the body's mass above its base of support. The muscles between the ribs and pelvis will need to react to these opposable motions rather than remaining rigid and braced. Might this be a good way to condition an area that is often the victim of isolated upper or lower body forces?

When the arm travels forward, the torso will rotate away from the arm. When the arm travels back, the torso will rotate toward the arm. The pelvis should be able to disassociate its movement from the torso and rotate in the opposite direction. If you struggle to rotate your rib cage to the right it might be a good idea to perform movements that encourage right rotation. That means performing a left arm horizontal press or a right arm horizontal row could achieve that goal.

When the hand rotates downward or inward, it is known as *pronation*. When it travels in the opposite direction it is known as *supination*. These two movements have the ability to dictate movement through the rest of the body. Pronation will cause the arm to internally rotate. This will drive the shoulder up and forward while encouraging the spine to flex.

Supination will create the opposite reaction. The arm will externally rotate. The shoulder will travel downward and retract and the spine will be encouraged to extend. Moving the hand and arm in various directions will provide the body with a myriad of movement experiences. This is encouraged to an even greater degree and also dependent upon the stance position. Bringing one leg forward will encourage the pelvis to rotate away from that leg. It could be a good idea to explore these variations in stances and movement combinations as it will provide the body with novelty and unique experiences, something the body and brain both thrive upon.

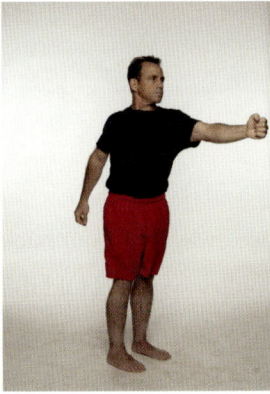

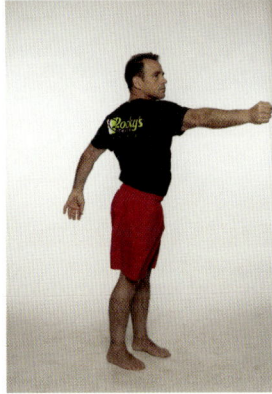

PRESSING

ONE-ARM CABLE LOW-TO-HIGH PRESS: Face away with your back toward the cable machine and use the low pulley system. Hold the cable handle in one hand with the cable between the forearm and rib cage. Press forward against the resistance of the cable to draw the arm away from the machine. Return the arm to the starting position. Allow the rib cage to rotate with the arm motion without leaning over.

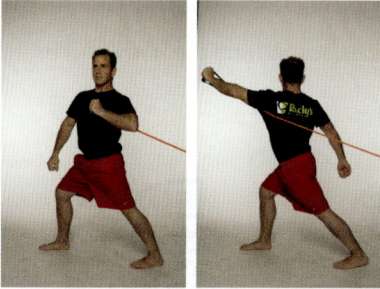

ONE-ARM HORIZONTAL CABLE PRESS WITH PRONATION: Face away with your back toward the cable machine and use the mid-level pulley system. Hold the cable handle in one hand with the cable between the forearm and rib cage. Press forward against the resistance of the cable to draw the arm away from the machine. Rotate the pressing hand internally so the thumb turns downward. Allow the spine to flex, feel the chest drop, and the rib cage rotate with the arm motion. Unwind the arm action and return to the starting position.

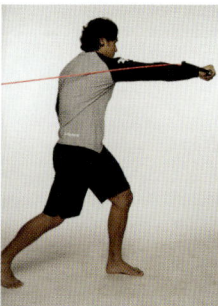

ONE-ARM HORIZONTAL CABLE PRESS WITH SUPINATION: Face away with your back toward the cable machine and use the mid-level pulley system. Hold the cable handle in one hand with the cable between the forearm and rib cage. Press forward against the resistance of the cable to draw the arm away from the machine. Rotate the pressing hand externally so the thumb turns

upward. Allow the spine to extend, feel the chest rise, and the rib cage rotate with the arm motion. Unwind the arm action and return to the starting position.

ONE-ARM OPPOSITE-SIDE ROTATIONAL OVERHEAD PRESS: Stand tall with feet parallel or with one leg forward. Reach one arm across, up, and around to the opposite side, above head height of the body. Return to center in a tall posture.

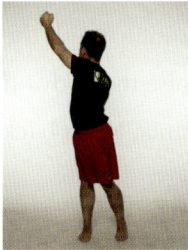

ONE-ARM OPPOSITE-SIDE SHOULDER PRESS: Stand tall with feet parallel or with one leg forward. Reach one arm off to the opposite side and above head height of the body. Allow the hips to travel in the opposite direction as the arm reaches sideways. Return to center in a tall posture.

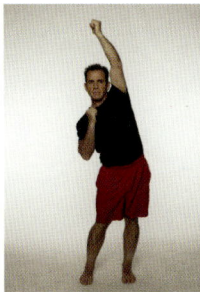

ONE-ARM SAME-SIDE ROTATIONAL OVERHEAD PRESS: Stand tall with feet parallel or with one leg forward. Reach one arm back and around to the same side, and above head height of the body. Return to center in a tall posture.

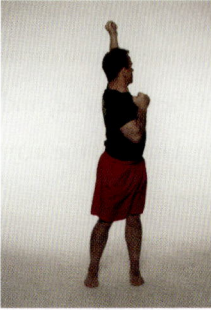

PUSH-UP: Lie face down on the floor, with hands outside the ribs, just below the shoulders. Ankles should be flexed so toes are in contact with the floor. Keep the body rigid as the arms press into, and raise the body off the floor until the arms are straight. In a controlled manner, lower back to the starting position.

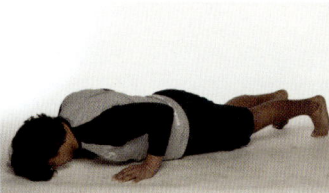

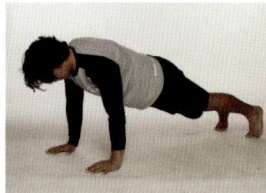

SHOULDER MATRIX

MOVEMENT #1: Stand tall with feet parallel or with one leg forward. Reach one arm forward at a time, and above head height of the body. Allow the hips to travel backward as the arm reaches forward. Return to center in a tall posture.

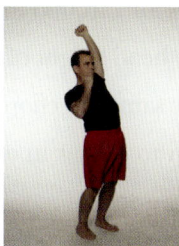

MOVEMENT #2: Stand tall with feet parallel or with one leg forward. Reach one arm backward at a time, and above head height of the body. Allow the hips to travel forward as the arm reaches backward. Return to center in a tall posture.

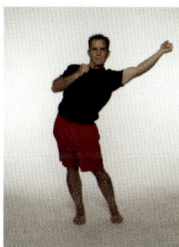

MOVEMENT #3: Stand tall with feet parallel or with one leg forward. Reach one arm off to the same side at a time, and above head height of the body. Allow the hips to travel in the opposite direction as the arm reaches sideways. Return to center in a tall posture.

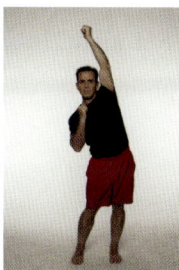

MOVEMENT #4: Stand tall with feet parallel or with one leg forward. Reach one arm off to the opposite side at a time, and above head height of the body. Allow the hips to travel in the opposite direction as the arm reaches sideways. Return to center in a tall posture.

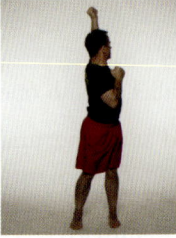

MOVEMENT #5: Stand tall with feet parallel or with one leg forward. Reach one arm back and around to the same side at a time, and above head height of the body. Allow the hips to travel in the same direction as the arm reaches sideways. Return to center in a tall posture.

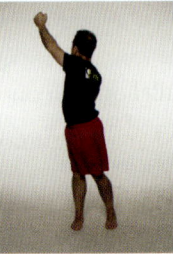

MOVEMENT #6: Stand tall with feet parallel or with one leg forward. Reach one arm across, up, and around to the opposite side at a time, and above head height of the body. Allow the hips to travel in the same direction as the arm reaches sideways. Return to center in a tall posture.

SHOULDER PRESS: Stand tall with feet parallel or in a forward split stance. Grip a barbell, or pair of dumbbells, in both hands, at shoulder height. Press the barbell up above the head until both arms are straight. In a controlled manner, lower the barbell back to the starting position.

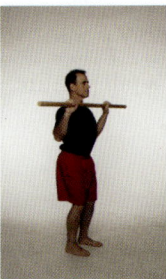

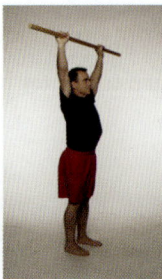

PULLING

ONE-ARM CABLE HORIZONTAL ROW: Face the cable machine and use the mid-level pulley system. Hold the cable handle in one hand. Reach forward and allow the cable to draw the arm toward the pulley. Hold firm and draw the elbow back to the side of the rib cage. Allow the rib cage to rotate with the arm motion. Return to the starting position.

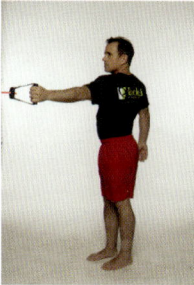

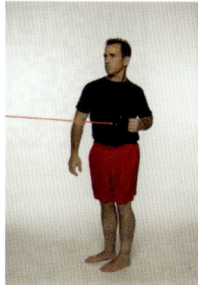

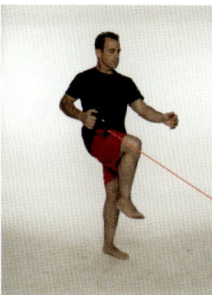

ONE-ARM CABLE LOW ROW: Face the cable machine and use the lower pulley system. Legs can be parallel, in a split stance, or for more challenge, balance on one leg. Hold the cable handle in one hand. Reach forward and allow the cable to draw the arm and torso toward the pulley. Hold firm and draw the elbow back to the side of the rib cage. Allow the rib cage to rotate with the arm motion. Return to the starting position.

ONE-ARM CABLE PULLDOWN: Face the cable machine and use the upper pulley system. Hold the cable handle in one hand. Reach forward and allow the cable to draw the arm upward toward the pulley. Hold firm and draw the elbow back to the side of the rib cage. Allow the rib cage to side bend and rotate with the arm motion. Return to the starting position.

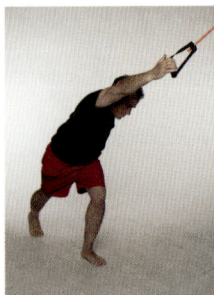

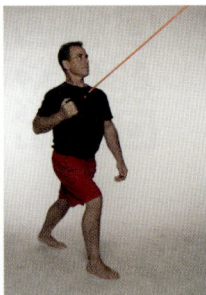

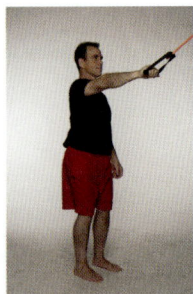

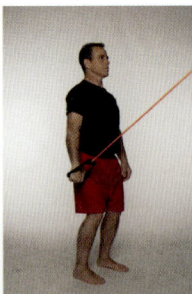

ONE-ARM CABLE STRAIGHT-ARM PULLDOWN: Face the cable machine and use the upper pulley system. Hold cable handle in one hand. Reach upward and allow the cable to draw the arm upward toward the pulley. Hold firm and draw the straight arm back to the side of the rib cage. Allow the rib cage to rotate with the arm motion. Return to the starting position.

FOUR-WAY OVERHEAD BAND PULL: A resistance band anchored at shoulder height, and held in one hand, is best used for the following movements:

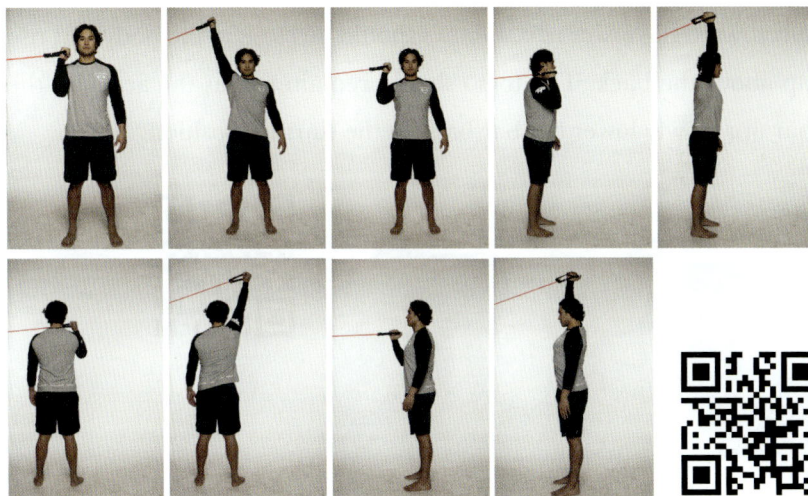

MOVEMENT #1: With the anchored end in front of the body, raise the arm straight up and down.

MOVEMENT #2: With the anchored end to the left side of the body, raise the arm straight up and down.

MOVEMENT #3: With the anchored end directly behind the body, raise the arm straight up and down.

MOVEMENT #4: With the anchored end to the right side of the body, raise the arm straight up and down.

BENT-OVER ROW: Stand tall with feet parallel and both hands holding a barbell. With a soft bend to the knees, hinge at the hips, lower the torso forward and down, so the shoulders are parallel with the hips. The bar should hang directly below the shoulders. Lift the barbell up so the bar lifts toward the lower ribs. Elbows should be close to the body and rise up above the back. The torso should remain still as the arms lift the bar up. Slowly lower the bar back to the starting position.

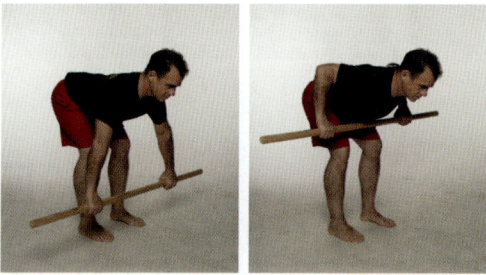

PULLDOWN: Grip a high pulley bar handle in both hands. Lower the body into a seated or squatting position, so arms are straight. Pull the bar down until it descends to chin level. Reverse directions back to the starting position.

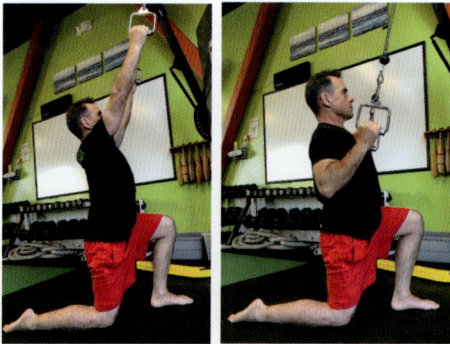

PULL-UP: Hang from a high bar with arms fully extended. Pull down on the bar to lift the body upward. Slowly lower back to a full hanging position before attempting another repetition.

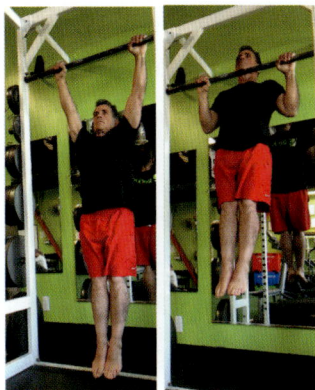

LEVEL CHANGES

LUNGES

A lunge is simply a stepping action away from center before returning back to center, or reestablishing a new center in the case of a walking lunge. The direction of a lunge dictates motion at the pelvis, hips, knees, ankles, and feet. A lunge also gets the legs to experience opposition with each other. One leg moves forward as the other stays behind. The body travels over one leg while it moves away from the other. In many ways, lunging could be considered an exaggeration of gait. This is all the more reason to incorporate such experiences into a conditioning program.

The action of the upper body during a lunge will dictate what occurs from the waist up, but can also govern how the lower body reacts. Traditionally, it has been encouraged to practice the lunge while maintaining a tall, balanced posture. This is great for focusing on proper leg mechanics and practicing how to balance the torso above the hips

> Over time, as the body endures long-term, repetitive actions under load, wear patterns begin to appear and the body is pulled away from its ideal center.

while moving through space. It would also be great to have the body experience a lunge when the torso is not balanced above the hips. Think of a tennis player sprinting across the court and reaching for a ball almost out of reach. What about when Grandpa has to catch the toddling grandson who leaned too far back in his chair? Lunging and reaching is an important athletic action that needs to be reinforced.

When one arm reaches overhead during a lunge, it can encourage the pelvis to move laterally in a couple of different ways. If the same-side arm of the lunging leg reaches upward, it would encourage the pelvis to sway toward that side. If it were the opposite arm reaching, it would encourage a lateral tilt away from that side. The same-side pelvis would hike while the opposite would drop. So, if you discovered through the dynamic assessment that it was challenging to hike one side of your pelvis, or sway to one side, you could encourage better mechanics by simply adding in the appropriate overhead action.

FRONT LUNGE: Stand tall with feet parallel. Step forward with one leg. Descend the body's weight onto the forward leg, bending into the hip and knee, while keeping the rear leg straight at the knee. Push off the front leg to return back to the starting position. Be sure not to allow the torso to lean forward or backward during the lunge. Maintain the head and shoulder position directly above the hips.

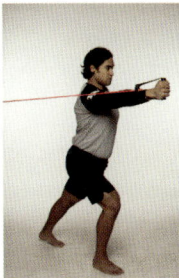

FRONT LUNGE WITH IPSILATERAL (SAME-SIDE ARM) HORIZONTAL PRESS: Stand tall with feet parallel while holding the handle of a resistance band or cable system in one hand. Step forward with one leg. Descend the body's weight onto the forward leg, bending into the hip and knee, while keeping the rear leg straight at the knee. At the same time, reach forward, at chest level, with the same-side arm as the stepping leg. Push off the front leg to return back to the starting position with arm retracted back to the side of the torso. Be sure not to allow the torso to lean forward or backward during the lunge. Maintain the head and shoulder position directly above the hips.

FRONT LUNGE WITH CONTRALATERAL (OPPOSITE-ARM) HORIZONTAL PRESS: Stand tall with feet parallel while holding the handle of a resistance band or cable system in one hand. Step forward with one leg. Descend the body's weight onto the forward leg, bending into the hip and knee, while keeping the rear leg straight at the knee. At the same time, reach forward, at chest level, with the opposite arm as the stepping leg. Push off the front leg to return back to the starting position with arm retracted back to the side of the torso. Be sure not to allow the torso to lean forward or backward during the lunge. Maintain the head and shoulder position directly above the hips.

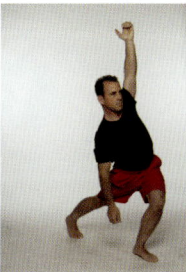

FRONT LUNGE WITH IPSILATERAL (SAME-SIDE ARM) OVERHEAD PRESS: Stand tall with feet parallel. Step forward with one leg. Descend the body's weight onto the forward leg, bending into the hip and knee, while keeping the rear leg straight at the knee. At the same time, reach upward overhead, with the same-side arm as the stepping leg. Push off the front leg to return back to the starting position with arm by the side. Be sure not to allow the torso to lean forward or backward during the lunge. Maintain the head and shoulder position directly above the hips.

FRONT LUNGE WITH CONTRALATERAL (OPPOSITE-ARM) OVERHEAD PRESS: Stand tall with feet parallel. Step forward with one leg. Descend the body's weight onto the forward leg, bending into the hip and knee, while keeping the rear leg straight at the knee. At the same time, reach upward overhead, with the opposite arm as the stepping leg. Push off the front leg to return back to the starting position with arm by the side. Be sure not to allow the torso to lean forward or backward during the lunge. Maintain the head and shoulder position directly above the hips.

BACK LUNGE: Stand tall with feet parallel. Step backward with one leg. Descend the body's weight onto the back leg, bending into the hip and knee, while keeping the front leg straight at the knee. Push off the back leg to return to the starting position. Be sure not to allow the torso to lean backward during the lunge.

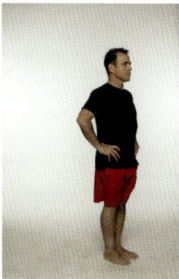

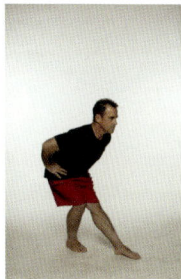

BACK LUNGE WITH IPSILATERAL (SAME-SIDE ARM) REACH: Stand tall with feet parallel. Step backward with one leg. Descend the body's weight onto the back leg, bending into the hip and knee, while keeping the front leg straight at the knee. Reach forward with the same-side arm as the forward leg. Allow the spine to flex or curl when reaching. Push off the back leg to return to the starting position. Be sure not to allow the torso to lean backward during the lunge.

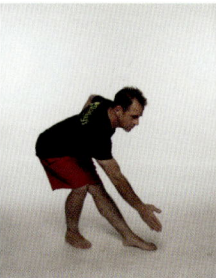

BACK LUNGE WITH CONTRALATERAL (OPPOSITE-ARM) REACH: Stand tall with feet parallel. Step backward with one leg. Descend the body's weight onto the back leg, bending into the hip and knee, while keeping the front leg straight at the knee and foot pointing up. Reach forward with the opposite arm as the forward leg. Allow the spine to flex or curl when reaching. Push off the back leg to return to the starting position. Be sure not to allow the torso to lean backward during the lunge.

DIAGONAL LUNGE: Stand tall with feet parallel. Step in a forward diagonal direction with one leg. Descend the body's weight onto the stepping leg, bending into the hip and knee, while keeping the trailing leg straight at the knee and allow the back heel to lift off the floor. Push off the stepping leg to return to the starting position. Be sure not to allow the torso to lean far forward or backward during the lunge.

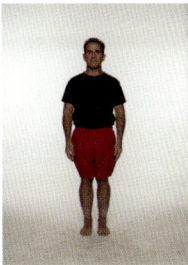

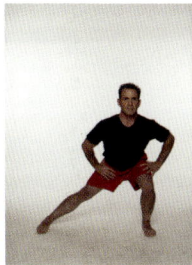

LATERAL LUNGE: Stand tall with feet parallel. Step sideways with one leg. Descend the body's weight onto the stepping leg, bending into the hip and knee, while keeping the trailing leg straight at the knee and foot flat on the floor. Push off the stepping leg to return to the starting position. Be sure not to allow the torso to lean far forward or backward during the lunge.

LATERAL LUNGE WITH IPSILATERAL (SAME-SIDE ARM) REACH: Stand tall with feet parallel. Step sideways with one leg. Descend the body's weight onto the stepping leg, bending into the hip and knee, while keeping the trailing leg straight at the knee and foot flat on the floor. Reach upward as high as possible, or downward with the same-side arm as the stepping leg. Push off the stepping leg to return to the starting position. Be sure not to allow the torso to lean far forward or backward during the lunge.

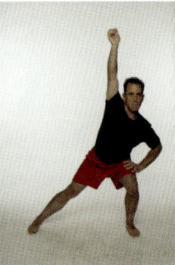

LATERAL LUNGE WITH CONTRALATERAL (OPPOSITE-ARM) REACH: Stand tall with feet parallel. Step sideways with one leg. Descend the body's weight onto the stepping leg, bending into the hip and knee, while keeping the trailing leg straight at the knee and foot flat on the floor. Reach upward as high as possible, or downward with the opposite arm as the stepping leg. Push off the stepping leg to return to the starting position. Be sure not to allow the torso to lean far forward or backward during the lunge.

LATERAL LUNGE WITH LATERAL OVERHEAD REACH AWAY: Stand tall with feet parallel. Step sideways with one leg. Descend the body's weight onto the stepping leg, bending into the hip and knee, while keeping the trailing leg straight at the knee and foot flat on the floor. Reach upward, and as high as possible, away from the stepping direction with both arms. Push off the stepping leg to return to the starting position. Be sure not to allow the torso to lean far forward or backward during the lunge.

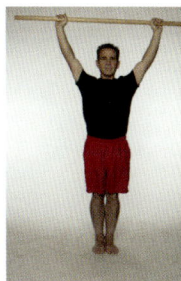

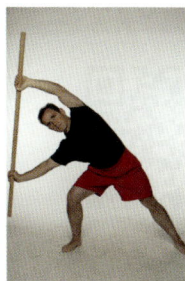

LATERAL LUNGE WITH LATERAL OVERHEAD REACH TOWARD: Stand tall with feet parallel. Step sideways with one leg. Descend the body's weight onto the stepping leg, bending into the hip and knee, while keeping the trailing leg straight at the knee and foot flat on the floor. Reach upward, and as high as possible, toward the stepping direction with both arms. Push off the stepping leg to return to the starting position. Be sure not to allow the torso to lean far forward or backward during the lunge.

ROTATIONAL LUNGE: Stand tall with feet parallel. Step back and to the same side with one leg in a rotating fashion. Descend the body's weight onto the stepping leg, bending into the hip and knee, while keeping the trailing leg straight at the knee and foot flat. Push off the stepping leg to return back to the starting position. Allow the torso to rotate around in the same direction during the lunge. Maintain the head and shoulder position directly above the hips.

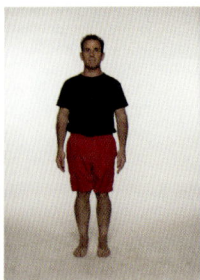

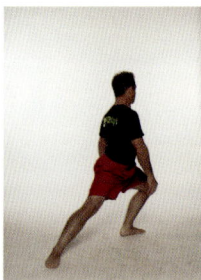

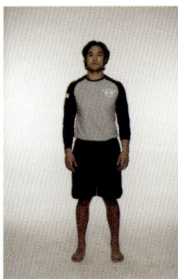

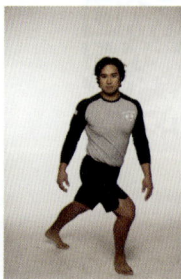

CROSSOVER LUNGE: Stand tall with feet parallel. Step forward and across to the opposite side with one leg. Descend the body's weight onto the forward leg, bending into the hip and knee, while keeping the rear leg straight at the knee. Push off the front leg to return to the starting position. Be sure not to allow the torso to lean forward or backward during the lunge. Maintain the head and shoulder position directly above the hips.

CROSSOVER LUNGE WITH CONTRALATERAL (OPPOSITE-ARM) REACH: Stand tall with feet parallel. Step forward and across to the opposite side with one leg. Descend the body's weight onto the forward leg, bending into the hip and knee, while keeping the rear leg straight at the knee. Reach upward as high as possible, or downward with the opposite arm as the stepping leg. Push off the front leg to return to the starting position. Be sure not to allow the torso to lean forward or backward during the lunge. Maintain the head and shoulder position directly above the hips.

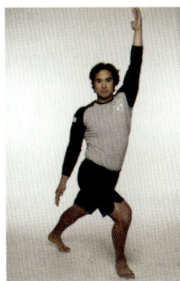

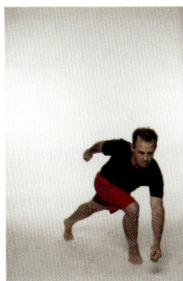

DEAD LIFTS

Dead-lifting movements are all about how to lift objects from the ground and return them down safely with control. Dead lifts are different from squats. During a squat the head and hips lift and lower at the same time and at the same rate. During a dead lift, the head lowers without the hips. The hips pivot or hinge to allow the pelvis to tilt forward on the journey down. It is common for people who have stiff hips, restricted pelvic motion, or who are unfamiliar with the motion, to flex into the lower back when lowering the upper body. This is an example of an improper lifting technique and should be avoided as it places undue strain and stress on the lower back. The pivotal point, or fulcrum, is the hip joint. As the torso lowers toward the floor to grab the weight, the hips flex and travel backwards. This allows the largest muscles of the body, the gluteals and hamstrings, to become the primary movers of the lift.

BENT-KNEE DEAD LIFT: Stand tall with feet parallel and knees softly bent. Keep the spine straight while hinging at the hips and bending at the knees. Lower the body until the thighs are parallel to the floor. The hips should pull backward during the descent, driving more weight into the heels. Reverse directions and return to the starting position.

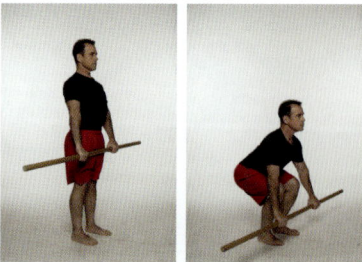

STRAIGHT LEG DEAD LIFT: Stand tall with feet parallel and knees softly bent. Keep the spine straight while hinging at the hips. Lower the torso until the back is parallel to the floor. The hips should pull backward as the torso descends, driving more weight into the heels. Reverse directions and return to the starting position.

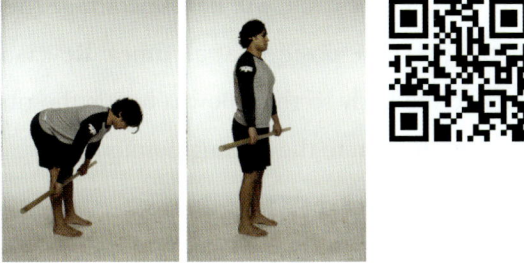

SINGLE LEG DEAD LIFT: Stand with feet parallel and knees softly bent. Lift one foot off the floor and reach backward with the leg as far as possible. By driving the leg back, the torso will automatically begin to lower forward. Maintain a straight spine position at all times. Reverse directions and return to the starting position.

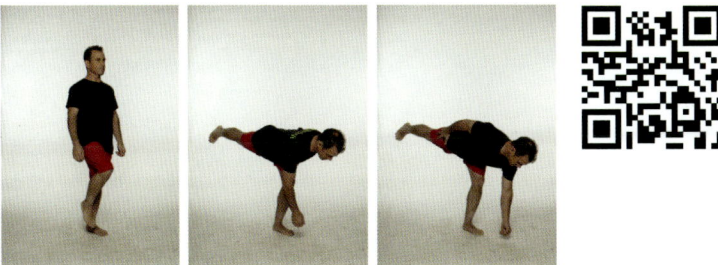

SINGLE LEG DEAD LIFT WITH ONE-ARM LOW ROW: Stand with feet parallel, knees softly bent, with one hand holding onto the handle of a low pulley or resistance band. Lift one foot off the floor and reach backward with the leg as far as possible. At the same time, allow the hand holding the handle to be pulled forward. By driving the leg back, the torso will automatically begin to lower forward and the band or cable will help encourage this action more. Maintain a straight spine position at all times. Reverse directions, pull the arm back to the body so the elbow is beside the rib cage at the top of the movement. Return to the starting position.

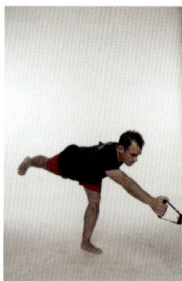

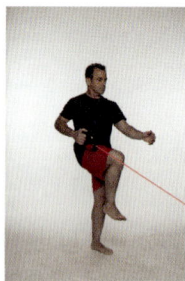

STEP-UPS

Fundamentally, a step-up is just a single leg squat that uses the opposite leg to assist with balance and stability. The direction of stepping can dictate what the hips and rest of the body experience. For instance, a traditional step-up (just like climbing stairs) will encourage one hip to experience flexion while the other leg experiences extension. The height of the step dictates the degree of hip flexion and extension. During a lateral step-up, one hip is encouraged to abduct while the other adducts. During a crossover step-up, one hip experiences a greater degree of rotation than the opposite hip. Incorporating movement and force in the upper body will encourage further action below. Depending on what is needed in someone's movement, patterns will help select which step-up to focus on.

STEP-UP: Stand behind a small box or bench. Take one foot and place it onto the box. Transfer the body's weight onto that leg and drive upward to a standing posture. Reverse directions and return to the starting position.

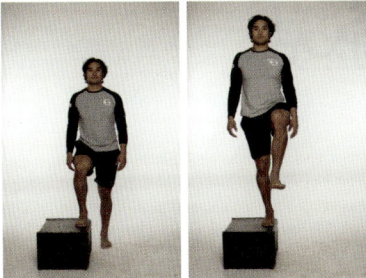

STEP-UP WITH CONTRALATERAL OVERHEAD PRESS: Stand behind a small box or bench. Take one foot and place it onto the box. Transfer the body's weight onto that leg and drive upward to a standing posture. Reverse directions and descend while reaching upward with the opposite arm of the pressing leg. Return to the starting position.

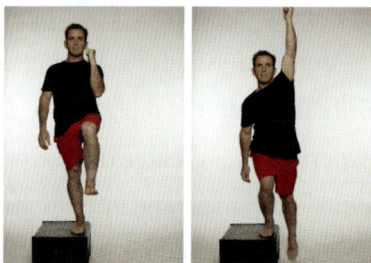

LATERAL STEP-UP: Stand beside a small box or bench. Place the foot closest to the box on top of the box. Transfer the body's weight laterally onto the box and drive upward to a standing posture. Reverse directions and return to the starting position.

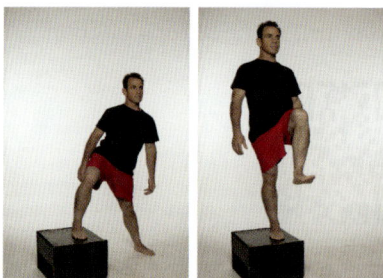

CROSSOVER STEP-UP: Stand beside a small box or bench. Take the outside leg and step across the body on to the box. Transfer the body's weight on to the box and drive upward to a standing posture. Reverse directions and return to the starting position.

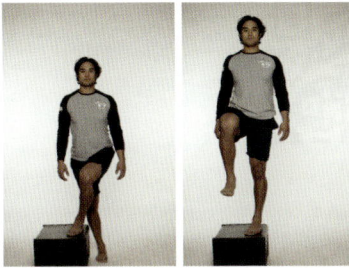

CROSSOVER STEP-UP WITH CONTRALATERAL (OPPOSITE-ARM) OVERHEAD REACH: Stand beside a small box or bench. Take the outside leg and step across the body onto the box. Transfer the body's weight onto the box and drive upward to a standing posture. Reverse directions and raise the opposite arm as the leg that is on the box. Return to the starting position.

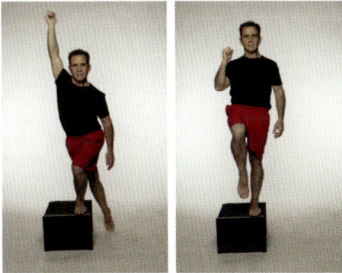

Remember that every action must add up to 100 percent no more and no less. Where you gain more movement, you have to lose it somewhere else and vice versa.

ROTATIONAL STEP-UP: Stand beside a small box or bench facing away. Place the foot closest to the box on top of the box. Transfer the body's weight laterally onto the box and drive upward in a rotating manner to a standing posture. Reverse directions and return to the starting position.

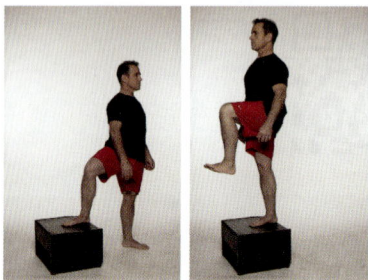

SQUATS

The squat is a movement that occurs in daily life. Every time a person sits they perform the squat. Considering how much sitting our society does, it makes sense to be good at squatting. Squatting is when the body is balanced over one or both feet. Foot positions may vary greatly because the legs can turn in and out, one foot can be forward of the other, and width may vary from narrow to very wide. The number of stance combinations add up to 27. This does not mean you would want to load a heavy barbell on the shoulders and begin squatting in 27 different ways. However, you may want to explore if your body is able to move in all the combinations while managing its bodyweight.

The difference between a squat and a lunge is that during a squat the feet, or foot, stays anchored to the ground while the body moves up and down within its base of support. A lunge is a stepping action that demands the body create a new base of support before returning back to center. During a squat, the head and hips lower at the same time and rate of speed. Other areas of the body also have an ideal way of managing the body's mass as it travels vertically.

The hips and pelvis begin the movement by flexing and tilting forward. In order to keep balanced over the feet the spine begins to extend and the shoulders retract with the shoulder blades. This will encourage the arms to externally rotate. Meanwhile, the femurs begin internally rotating and the knees move toward each other as they flex. The ankles begin dorsiflexing and the feet drop into pronation. As the body begins its journey back to a tall, standing posture the joints reverse directions and the opposite of what is described above occurs. As greater amounts of weight are applied to the body, some of these joint actions may need to change. Knees are encouraged to minimize the motion toward each other and reducing foot pronation is often coached.

SINGLE LEG SQUAT WITH GLIDING BACK FOOT: Stand tall with feet parallel. Place all of the body's weight onto one leg. Slide the other leg back behind the body and slightly across to the opposite side as far as possible (this movement may be better executed with the sliding foot resting on a plastic furniture mover or a wax paper plate). The back foot should be able to easily lift off the floor throughout the entire movement. Reach forward or downward with the same-side arm as the back foot. Attempt to create as much distance between the reaching hand and the sliding foot. Allow the torso to lower and turn in the direction of the forward leg. Reverse directions and return to the starting position.

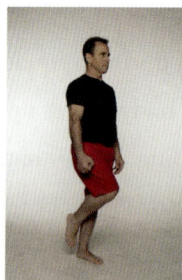

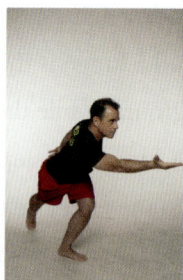

SPLIT SQUAT: Begin this exercise in a half-kneeling position with one knee resting on the floor directly below the hip joint, and the opposite leg forward with the foot flat and the knee at a right angle. Maintain a tall posture so the head is above the shoulders, and the shoulders are above the hips. Press evenly with both legs to rise vertically in a straight line. Keep the tall posture at all times on the ascent and the descent back to the starting position.

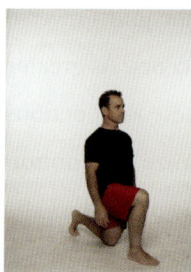

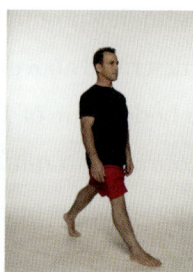

SPLIT SQUAT WITH REAR LEG RAISED: Begin this exercise in a half-kneeling position with one knee resting on the floor directly below the hip joint with the roof of the foot resting behind the body on a box, and the opposite leg forward with the foot flat and the knee at a right angle. Maintain a tall posture so the head is above the shoulders, and the shoulders are above the hips. Press through the forward leg to rise vertically in a straight line. Keep the tall posture at all times on the ascent and the descent back to the starting position.

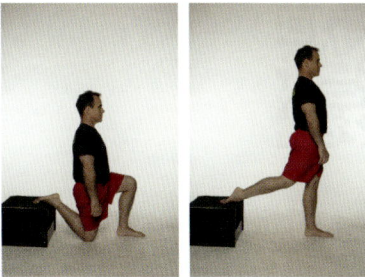

SPLIT SQUAT WITH CONTRALATERAL (OPPOSITE-ARM) OVERHEAD PRESS: Begin this exercise in a half-kneeling position with one knee resting on the floor directly below the hip joint, and the opposite leg forward with the foot flat and the knee at a right angle. Maintain a tall posture so the head is above the shoulders, and the shoulders are above the hips. Press evenly with both legs to rise vertically in a straight line. Keep the tall posture at all times on the ascent. As the body descends back to the starting position, raise the opposite arm of the forward leg up overhead.

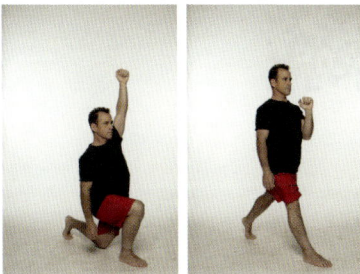

SPLIT SQUAT WITH IPSILATERAL (SAME-SIDE ARM) OVERHEAD PRESS: Begin this exercise in a half-kneeling position with one knee resting on the floor directly below the hip joint, and the opposite leg forward with the foot flat and the knee at a right angle. Maintain a tall posture so the head is above the shoulders, and the shoulders are above the hips. Press evenly with both legs to rise vertically in a straight line. Keep the tall posture at all times on the ascent. As the body descends back to the starting position, raise the same-side arm of the forward leg up overhead.

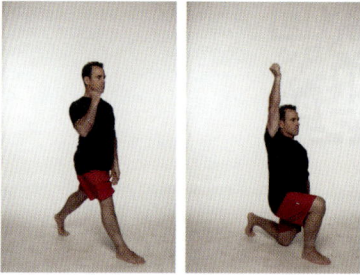

SQUAT: Stand tall with feet parallel. Bend at the hips and then knees as the body lowers into a seated-like position. Ideally the hips should descend until parallel with the knees. Reverse directions and return to the starting position. Head and torso will travel forward slightly but should remain back behind the knees and not over or in front.

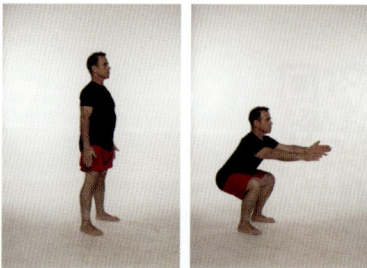

SQUAT WITH BILATERAL PULL: Stand tall with feet parallel while holding the cable or resistance band handles in each hand. Bend at the hips and then knees, as the body lowers into a seated-like position while the arms reach forward. Ideally, the hips should descend until parallel with the knees, and the arms should be fully extended at the elbows. Head and torso will travel forward slightly, but should remain back behind the knees and not over or in front. Reverse directions and return to the starting position as the arms pull the handles to the side of the ribs.

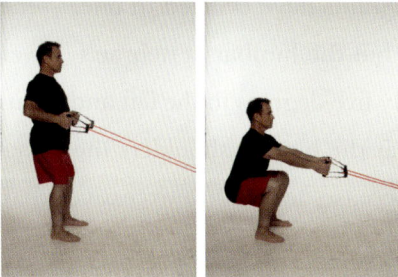

ROTATION

Most muscles responsible for locomotion do not attach in a simple vertical or horizontal direction. They are attached in a more diagonal manner. So, when these muscles lengthen or shorten they create a rotational action to that area of the body. The amount of rotation really depends on the area of the body and the body's position. If it occurs at the right place with the proper timing, all is good. If it occurs somewhere else or at the wrong time, the potential for harm is great. For instance, the hip and shoulder joints have evolved to offer some of the greatest degrees of rotation but the lumbar vertebrae's (lower back) capacity for rotation is roughly five degrees to the left and right. If there is a reduction of rotation at the hips or shoulders the lower back's rotation may attempt to increase, leading to excessive wear and/or injury.

Stance dictates degree of pelvic rotation. When standing with feet parallel, the pelvis should have an equal amount of rotation to the left and right. When one leg is forward of the other, the pelvis naturally rotates away from the forward leg. The pelvis can rotate toward the forward leg but the range will be restricted and if more rotation is needed it will demand more often from other areas. As discussed in the previous Pressing & Pulling section, arm movement will often dictate rib rotation. The driving arm dictates which PNF paths (the cross-body connective tissues that run from one shoulder to the opposite hip) engage.

ONE-ARM CABLE ROTATION-FORWARD: Hold the handle of a resistance band or pulley system in one hand. Pull the band or cable across the body. Be sure to allow the rib cage to rotate in the same direction as the handle. Return to the starting position.

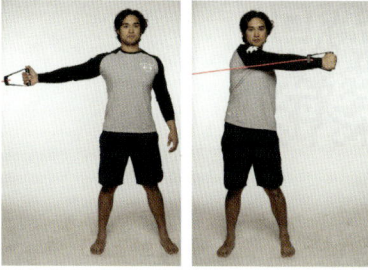

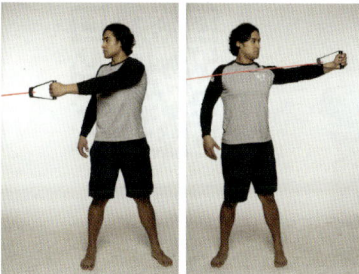

ONE-ARM CABLE ROTATION-BACKWARD: Hold the handle of a resistance band or pulley system in one hand. Turn the body so the band is crossed in front of the body. Pull the band or cable across the body. Be sure to allow the rib cage to rotate in the same direction as the handle. Return to the starting position.

CABLE ROTATION-DRIVING ACROSS: Hold the handle of a resistance band or pulley system in both hands. Pull the band or cable across the body. Be sure to allow the rib cage to rotate in the same direction as the handle. Return to the starting position.

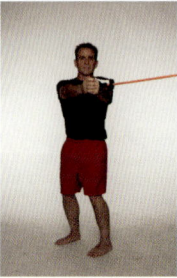

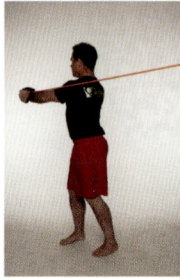

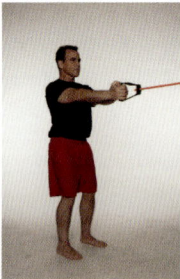

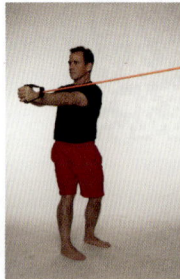

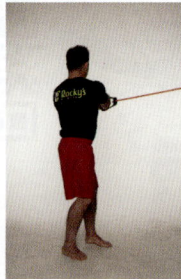

CABLE ROTATION-PULLING BACK: Face the pulley or anchor point of a resistance band. Hold the handle of a resistance band or pulley system in both hands. Pull the band back behind the body. Be sure to allow the rib cage to rotate in the same direction as the handle. Return to the starting position.

PLANK CLOCK: Support the body face down on the floor with the hands and feet (for less intensity the knees may be supportive instead of the feet). Imagine the body is positioned in the center of a giant clock with the head pointing to 12 o'clock and the feet toward 6 o'clock. Reach with one hand as far as possible toward 12 o'clock. Repeat with the opposite hand. Continue this alternating reaching action around the imaginary clock at every hour until all hours have been touched. Allow the body to move as the arm reaches rather than maintain a rigid, board-like posture.

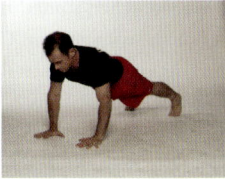

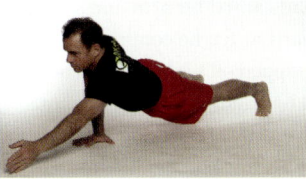

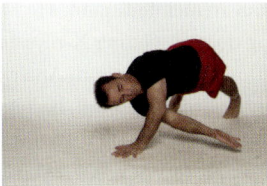

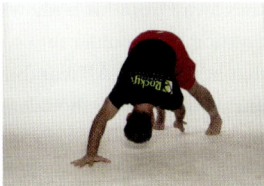

TARGET THE PROBLEM, NOT THE SYMPTOM: FROZEN SHOULDER

A local surfer came in to see me about an injury he had sustained while out on the waves. He told me that he had been surfing on a pretty big day and got thrown off his board. During his constant tumbling in the white wash his hand got caught in the reef. His forward momentum had caused his arm and shoulder to get wrenched something awful. Being the true die-hard surfer, he continued to surf after the heavy wipeout. On his very next wave his foot slipped off his board and he wrenched his knee. That was the end of his surf session and he paddled gingerly to shore.

The weeks that followed were filled with pain and immobility. Although his knee slowly recovered from the wrenching, his shoulder did not. He found he could not lift his arm more than a couple of inches away from his body without tremendous pain. He had spent the next few months resting his shoulder and seeing doctors, getting X-rays and MRIs. The diagnosis was that he had a SLAP tear (Superior Labral tear from Anterior to Posterior). That is when the cartilage in his shoulder joint, called the labrum, becomes torn. The doctor's recommendation was to perform surgery. The surgeon would go into his shoulder joint and remove the torn-away tissue and, if possible, sew the tears together. After the surgery he would need several weeks of physical therapy and it would be months before he could even consider putting on a wetsuit.

The injured surfer was encouraged by a friend to make an appointment with me just to see if there was another approach to try before going in for surgery. In the months since his surf accident, with the help of a physical therapist, he had been able to increase his range of motion to the point that he could lift his arm to shoulder height with minimal pain. When he attempted to reach higher he found the pain increased and would not allow him to go any further. There was no more improvement after that.

When we met, I took him through an assessment. What we discovered was that his shoulder blade moved quicker and more than it needed. This meant somewhere else was not moving enough. Remember, the body's overall movement adds up to 100 percent, no more, no less. We discovered his hips were not moving enough to assist in reaching the arm upward. His spine was not side bending or rotating enough to encourage proper motion, either. In essence his frame was on lock-down, pulling him in the direction of the fetal position. It was bracing to protect from further pain and injury.

We began to "interview" his body. What would happen if we got the hips and spine to move a little more? What would it feel like if we were to slow down the motion of the shoulder blade? What positions could he move into that were pain-free? We let his body inform us as to how to move and how much. Some pretty cool things began to happen; within a matter of minutes he could raise his arm over his head without pain. He had been unable to perform this action for over six months! By listening to what his body told us we were able to create a strategy of motion that unlocked areas that were in a constant, unyielding loop of fear and immobility.

A couple of weeks later he returned for another session and his range of motion had continued to improve. However, there were still areas of pain or discomfort that occurred when his arm moved in certain directions. After listening to what the body was telling us, we did a few more movements and also began working with Indian clubs. In just five minutes of swinging the clubs in certain patterns his jaw dropped. He could feel how his shoulder had released its tension and the movements that caused pain no longer did. It really is almost like magic when you see how the body can improve and heal itself when you listen to what it has to tell you. Perhaps somewhere down the road he might need to get surgical attention for the wear and tear his lifestyle creates. Or maybe not. He seems to be doing quite well on the waves without it.

CHAPTER 8
PUTTING IT ALL TOGETHER

Now that you have read through the chapters addressing soft tissue rehydration (a.k.a. foam rolling), assessing and reassessing, mobility drills, and strength exercises, it is time to create your program. This final chapter will provide you more insight to the various elements that make up your routine. You may be asking yourself questions such as: How often should I perform the routine? Which exercises and drills should I be doing? How much weight should I be using? How much time is involved with the routine? The answers to these and other questions can be found below.

The ultimate goal of this program is for you to develop a strong, fully functioning body. Continually assessing and reassessing what state your body is in will act as your guide or compass. In this book, we've used the simple, yet at the same time incredibly complex, act of walking, the most common, universal movement of all, and which has been engrained in humans for millions of years, to determine the exercise selection. All the movement assessments are basic biomechanics, which should normally occur at some point in the gait cycle. If there are movements missing, or are challenging to perform, that lets us know where to begin and what to try and improve. The program is an exploration into the body, and enables you to understand what it needs. The body (and autonomic nervous system) will guide you in designing a program that will benefit you in the moment, in real time. (And for you trainers reading this book, it will help guide you in designing programs for clients.) More may be revealed as you work to improve your strength, posture, balance, structural alignment, etc., and as you restore better movement, increase strength, and eliminate some compensations. Do not be surprised if older compensations may begin to appear. This is like peeling back the onion layers to get to the core. You may find that movement patterns you have developed over the years originated from the effects of an injury, surgery, or accident you sustained at a very early age. So, it is really a process rather than a one-time thing.

As I've stressed throughout this book, all movement requires strength and mobility. How much strength and how much mobility is dependent on several factors: nervous system, past experiences, injuries, surgeries, accidents, emotional state, hormonal balance, etc. The conventional approach to strength training accomplishes the goal of increased strength in one major way: apply resistance to build the size of the muscle fibers to produce greater degrees of force and power. The time involved for muscles to increase in size is measured in weeks. Although this approach has proven to be incredibly effective, and tremendous amounts of time and research have been devoted to improving it every year, it does come at a price. Over time, as the body endures long-term, repetitive actions under load, wear patterns begin to appear and the body is pulled away from its ideal center. These patterns, combined with subtle structure distortions, muscular imbalances, and compensatory actions, will increase the likelihood of injuries and corrective surgeries somewhere down the road.

It is not so much the exercise as it is the degree to which each exercise is appropriate for you. It is imperative, for long-term strength and full body function, that the exercises be the ones you need at that period of time. Exercises should help promote balance among all of the muscles, alignment of all joints, and the most efficient flow of energy through the entire body. The time involved to changing the nervous system to increase strength levels in the body is measured in seconds. It would be so much better if we were to combine both of these powerful approaches to increase muscular size while unlocking restricted movement, improving joint function, enhancing muscular balance, and reducing the likelihood of injury.

ASSESSING THROUGH NEUROLOGICAL RESPONSE

The all-governing nervous system is the best barometer to use when determining which movements to encourage, how much intensity to use, and how long to work. It is the subconscious portion which controls body functions like breathing, heart rate, blood flow, blood pressure, and digestion. It also regulates balance, movement, strength, coordination, and mobility. It does this through two types of responses or reactions. The type of response is dictated primarily by how the central nervous system receives and interprets stimuli from inside and outside the body. The responses are known as the *sympathetic* and *parasympathetic* nervous system. The sympathetic system prepares the body for exercise by increasing heart rate, blood pressure, and respiration. However, the sympathetic system also responds to stimuli which are interpreted as threats. Pain, injuries, strains, muscular imbalance, distorted posture, illness, trauma, and surgeries have the potential to be interpreted as threats to the nervous system. If the sympathetic response is too strong, it will reduce movement, redirect blood flow, restrict muscular length, and decrease muscular strength. These reactions are, of course, counterproductive to improving strength and overall fitness.

It is the parasympathetic system that wants to be encouraged when training. The parasympathetic response will elevate strength levels, improve joint motion, and increase balance and coordination. When the sympathetic system is overactive, it is the parasympathetic system that needs to activate more in order to inhibit the fight or flight response.

It is by continually assessing and reassessing that we learn which response is governing body functions at any given moment. There may be times, when reassessing, when no change is experienced. This could simply mean that there were not enough stimuli to create a response in either direction. Try altering some element of the drill or exercise, and reassess to see if that triggers a response. Or, if there is an ideal balance between the sympathetic and parasympathetic systems.

ELEMENTS TO ALTER COULD BE:

Action: Drills or exercise selection

Duration: Time under tension

Range of motion: Full or partial

Tempo: Slow, medium, or fast

Progression: Unassisted, assisted, or resisted

Load: Light, medium, heavy

DRILLS & EXERCISE SELECTION

Your selection of mobility and strength exercises will be based on the results of your assessment. The important thing to remember is that everybody is unique and that means that some exercises in one column of the strength and mobility charts (found in the Appendix) will not have the same effect as others. The selection of exercises in each column stems from how the joints of the body relate to one another when the body is in motion. Because people move differently, it is impossible to design one perfect program for everyone. Your body will be the teacher and guide. You are able to use any or all of the three assessments to determine which movements to place in your program. Out of the ten movement assessments found in Chapter 3, choose one or two which were the most challenging, or that felt as if they were missing, compared to the opposite side or direction. You will find that the movement assessments correlate to each of the 8 body shapes and the 7 foot pressures. Not every person will fall cleanly into one category but may be a combination of different body shapes. Refer to the columns on the mobility, strength, and soft tissue charts (found in the Appendix) that match the selected movements, shapes, and pressures. There are many drills and exercises under each column. It is not imperative, nor is it intended, that you perform every one of them (or that your client perform every one of them). Simply choose between three and ten from the mobility charts and the same number from the strength chart.

Perform one of the mobility drills and reassess to see if it helped. If it did, keep that drill in your routine for a little while. If it did not help, move on to another drill in the column. Continue in this fashion until you have several effective drills in your workout "toolkit." You can rotate through these drills for a few workouts or a few weeks. You will begin to feel, more and more, the effect they create in your structure and soft tissue. There should be a sense of strength and freedom of movement, a lightness or floating feeling—the

> Because people move differently, it is impossible to design one perfect program for everyone. Your body will be the teacher and guide.

opposite of feeling compressed and heavy. When you begin the program, it is a good idea to reassess after every drill so you can create a better sense of how the body responds (sympathetically or parasympathetically). After a while, you will almost instantly be able to predict the outcome of the reassessment and know which of the two responses will show.

Perform one of the strength exercises on the chart in the appropriate column and reassess to see if that helped. If it did, choose more exercises from this list. If it didn't help, go down the list and choose another. If you progress through the top column and still have not found the appropriate exercises, choose from the bottom column. Remember that some areas of the body respond better to moving the body in the direction it moves well, while other areas respond better to moving the body in the direction in which it moves poorly. Continue with this process until you have several strength exercises in your arsenal. You can use these exercises for just the one workout, or you can keep them in your routine for a few workouts or a few weeks. Be sure to develop a new program at least once a month if you train three times per week or more.

Like the mobility drills, be sure to reassess after each exercise, at least initially. It will help get you more connected with your body and get a better sense of which autonomic response it triggers. The number of possible strength exercises are virtually limitless, but there is only so much room in one book. This means that there are countless exercises that have the potential to provide a positive or negative response. Feel free to go outside of the suggested list if you choose. Exercise is meant to be an exploration in movement to find your strengths and weaknesses and improve upon them. In some cases, it may take a few workouts to home in on the best movements for you to practice.

> Exercise is meant to be an exploration in movement, to find your strengths and weaknesses and improve upon them.

After every workout, or at least from time to time, perform the ten movement assessments, the posture assessment, and check in to see where your foot pressure resides to see how the body is changing. As you become more familiar with the assessments, they should only take a few minutes to perform and this "check in" might provide you with even more insight. Do not be surprised if you feel even more off balance. The possible reason for this is that your subconscious mind has considered where your body has been positioned as balanced and "normal." When the body shifts closer to center it may seem like this "new normal" is far from where the old center was. Over a short amount of time the new center will normalize, and the brain will organize movement around it.

IF NOT ONE, THEN THE OTHER

As stated above, if you find that one column (the structural column) in a chart is not giving you the positive, desired response, choose exercises from the sister column (the functional column). If not one, then the other. There are really only two choices for the body, this way or that. Most of the time one will provide a different outcome than the other. This is based on the first two rules of *Anatomy in Motion*: Rule No. 1: Muscles lengthen before they contract, and Rule No. 2: Joints act, muscles react.

A simple example of the difference between the two is determining what to do with a pronated foot that remains flat at the medial arch and has difficulty creating an arch. The first rule would encourage the foot to pronate even more beyond its normalized flatness, so the lengthened muscles under the arch experience even more length, and then react by shortening, thus driving the medial arch to a higher and more neutral position. The second rule would act to drive the flattened arch into the high, lifted position it has trouble getting into. This way the shortened muscles on the outside edge and roof of the foot, which have trouble lengthening, will be encouraged to get longer. It is one way or the other. There really isn't any other choice. Some areas of the body will do better with one approach compared to the other.

SOFT TISSUE HYDRATION/SELF-MYOFASCIAL RELEASE

Think of soft tissue hydration as the cheapest form of massage you will ever find. What a great way to start and finish your routine! The true purpose of rolling, pressing, and releasing pressure against the body is to improve circulation throughout soft tissue that needs it. Use the foot map to determine what areas to target, or choose from the list of target areas which appear next to the strength and mobility charts for your body shape or missing movement. Time spent on rehydration may vary from one person to the next. The frequency can be as often as several times a day or just during the workouts.

MOVEMENT PROGRESSION

Progressions can occur over any length of time such as days, weeks, or months. It depends upon how the body responds to the movements and what the reassessment tells you. For those who have very few limitations or imbalances, the progression could actually occur within the workout itself. The first set could be unilateral, the second set could be alternating actions, and the third set could be bilateral motions. Everyone is different and there is not one size which fits all. Movement progressions can also range from simple to complex. When performing most of the movements in this book it is best to begin with simple, and progress to more complex motions.

For instance, if one of the strength exercises on your

list is a left leg front lunge with same-side overhead press, it is best to work on the lunge mechanics before incorporating the arm action. Or begin with the arm action before incorporating the lunge mechanics. Simple to complex. If, when performing any exercise, it feels like it is too complex, just reduce the number of limbs moving and focus on where the body is meant to travel before returning to center. As it becomes more comfortable, add back in more complexity. Remember, your

> Just because you do not use a dumbbell does not mean you are not strength training. The weight of the body may be an adequate amount of resistance and may not require more in the form of dumbbells, barbells, cables, etc.

autonomic system will be able to guide you to know if it is too simple or too complex based on the response you receive. Here is a simple guide when it comes to movement. Focus on one side of the body before performing alternating actions or bilateral motions.

MOVEMENT PROGRESSIONS:

- Unilateral (working one side or one motion)
- Alternating (taking turns between one side or one motion with each repetition or set)
- Bilateral (moving both sides of the body in the same direction at the same time)

LOAD PROGRESSION

How much resistance, or intensity, is needed varies from one exercise to the next. There are some movements where the body is strongest and may require tremendous load to challenge the muscles. Meanwhile, there are many more movements where much less resistance is needed and a person's body weight may be too much. Just because you do not use a dumbbell does not mean you are not strength training. The weight of the body may be an adequate amount of resistance and may not require more in the form of dumbbells, barbells, cables, etc. Ask any gymnast. The average weight of an arm is 5 percent to 6 percent of total body weight. A 150-pound person's arms weigh about 8 pounds each. The legs are about 18 percent of total body weight. That means each leg weighs 27 pounds on that 150-pound person. The trunk is about 54 percent of body weight, and thus would weigh about 80 pounds. The head is an additional 8 to 10 pounds. Thus, the weight of your body can often be enough to really pose a challenge to muscles. It is very important to be able to move well before adding additional resistance. There are also movements for which additional resistance or even body weight may be too much and some form of assistance may be required to accomplish the action. It is essential that you establish a level of progression when performing the exercises. To simplify matters we will just use three levels of load progression. From easiest to hardest they are:

Assisted: Giving the body assistance in accomplishing the action. This can be in the form of holding onto a countertop, using dowels to support, changing the angle of the body relative to gravity, or any way that reduces bodyweight resistance so the action is successful.

Unassisted: Not using any assistance or external resistance (dumbbells, bands, etc.), but simply using the body's weight as the level of resistance. Ideally, a person should be able to support their own bodyweight while moving through space in all directions.

Resisted: The use of additional external resistance (dumbbells, medicine balls, barbells, cables, kettlebells, etc.) when the body's weight is not an ample level of resistance for a given exercise.

The success of your movement and how the autonomic nervous system responds to the exercise will let you know if you are at the proper level of resistance, or if you need to regress to a lower intensity or progress to more intensity. Do not be surprised if the level of intensity varies from one workout to the next. Remember, the body is continually adapting to its environment; depending on what occurs between workouts will affect strength levels every time. There will be days when you are not feeling as strong as the day before and it will be easier to adjust your level of intensity. Then there will be days where you feel good but the autonomic nervous system is informing you the same level of resistance you were using during your last workout is too much for this workout. It is important to listen to your subconscious. It does not have the capacity to lie. It is simply receiving, interpreting, and responding to everything you experience, even if you are not consciously aware of it. During those times, lower the intensity level and get to work.

FREQUENCY

How many times should you follow this program? It really depends. There is no magic number. I would suggest that performing the routine a minimum of two days per week to bring about some change. Typically, the more frequent, the more changes will occur. However, too much of anything is not necessarily a good thing. Rely on what the brain tells you. It is, after all, your best guide. A number is just a number. Some time ago, an exercise physiologist made an unsupported claim that a person should not exercise the same muscle groups every day, and that 24 hours of rest, in between training the same area, was necessary. It was a blanket statement designed to prevent overtraining, but it somehow became the golden rule for decades, without anyone questioning it. Truth be told, the frequency of workouts will vary from one person to the next and should be based on how your brain and body respond in the moment.

If there is one element which the majority of people could perform every day it is the mobility portion of this program. This is especially the case if the mobility drills are varied from one day to the next, since the body experiences a variety of demands constantly. The strength exercises may be a different story. Depending on the level of intensity of the strength workout, it might be good to allow a day of rest in between sessions every now and then. Regardless of the frequency, getting proper amounts of sleep in between workouts is essential for good repair and strength gains.

PROGRAM OPTIONS

The body is continually adapting to its environment and the demands placed upon it from one minute to the next. This is why it might be beneficial to adjust your workout routine often to address the constant change. If a routine becomes too tedious, then a new program every week or month can also produce positive outcomes. The frequency with which you change the training program is up to you and your nervous system. For many, it will be all about personal preference and how far down the rabbit hole you're willing to travel.

Here are three potential approaches to take:

1. Assess the body with every workout and choose which movements it needs from the charts provided.
2. Assess the body every week to develop a weekly routine.
3. Assess the body every month to develop a monthly routine

VOLUME

The volume of work refers to how many sets and repetitions of each exercise or drill you should perform. To some degree, this is based on personal preference and how much time you are able to or want to devote to improving your movements. Of course, if the volume is too low, the likelihood of seeing much change is also low. Likewise, if the volume is too high, it might create a threat response and be counterproductive to seeing improvement. As a general rule, most people will benefit from a program comprised of an equal amount of mobility drills and strength exercises. Then there will be those others who require more mobility while others need more strength. It is really dependent on your individual needs.

This does not mean that people who consider themselves weak should focus more attention on strength exercises compared to mobility. It could be that their low strength levels are more related to their degree of mobility. As stated in previous chapters, when joints are "jammed" or lacking mobility, the autonomic nervous system emits a sympathetic response and lowers overall strength levels. Therefore, giving the body the experience of mobility, in the correct regions, will instantly improve strength levels, at times more than any strength exercise could. This also does not mean that people who have been told or who consider themselves "hypermobile" do not need mobility, because they do. It may not be in the areas with abundant motion, but there are other places yearning for it. Those who have more mobility in some joints of their body will also have joints somewhere else that do not have enough. It is a matter of physics and biomechanics. Remember that every action must add up to 100 percent, no more and no less. Where you gain more movement, you have to lose it somewhere else and vice versa.

When it comes to volume of work, here are some basic guidelines to use:

Soft tissue hydration

- Select 2 to 4 regions to work on.
- Average number of sets: 1 to 2.
- Average number of repetitions: 5 to 15.
- Increase depth of pressure as tolerated.

Strength exercises

- Select 3 to 6 exercises.
- Average number of sets: 1 to 3.
- Average number of repetitions: 5 to 15.
- Begin with low repetitions so new movements do not fatigue and new compensatory patterns develop.
- Increase repetition range based on the central nervous system response.

Mobility drills

- Select 3 to 6 drills.
- Number of sets: 1 to 2.
- Number of repetitions may vary between 5 to 20.
- Explore end ranges of motion in a pain-free environment.
- Increase range of motion as mobility improves and based on central nervous system response.

PAIN

Pain, although it is not a nice feeling, provides us with information. Pain could be telling you that the body's structural alignment is not in a place where that movement will be beneficial. Pain could mean that the coordinated effort is not ideal, or the form is incorrect. Pain could be letting you know that the load is too great and the body has trouble handling it safely. It could mean a host of other things, too. Pain is the way the subconscious part of the brain can communicate with the conscious part. It is much like a crying baby. The baby does not have the ability to use words to let us know it is hungry, or needs a diaper change, or just wants to be held. Crying is the baby's way of getting your attention. Pain is the same way. Unfortunately, many people do not pay attention to pain. They just let the baby in their brain keep crying and crying. When the brain experiences pain, or more to the point, threat, it responds by restricting joint range of motion, increasing muscular tension, reducing force potential, compromising balance and coordination, and decreasing visual acuity. Then there are all of the other things a threat response can bring on, such as increased resting heart rate and blood pressure, impaired digestion, reduced circulation, and decreased respiration. This is why moving into pain or worse yet, living in pain, is not a good idea.

Pain comes in many forms. Pain can be a sharp sensation in the joint, a nagging ache in the soft tissue, or a throbbing headache. There are many more ways which pain can express itself. It is not always a flashing neon sign, it could be at a low-grade level such as itchiness. No matter how it appears, when it comes to pain it is a simple yes or no. There is no "kind of," or "just a little." If someone asks you if you feel pain, it is either yes or no. If you shrug your shoulders, that means yes. If you squint or make some facial expression, that means yes. If you rub a sore area after an exercise, that means yes. If you have

> When the brain experiences pain, or more to the point - threat, it responds by restricting joint range of motion, increasing muscular tension, reducing force potential, compromising balance and coordination, and decreasing visual acuity.

to pause and think about it, that means yes. A no answer comes quickly and without thinking about it. It is clear, concise, and certain. Anything less than that is usually a yes. So, here are some bullet points that you can consider as basic guidelines when it comes to pain:

- Do not move into pain!
- Stop that movement!
- Check to see if your form is correct.
- Reduce the level of resistance and see if pain persists.
- Reduce the range of motion if the pain occurred at the end range.
- Change the tempo of the movement and see if pain persists.
- Do not perform the movement for the time being if pain persists.

TARGET THE PROBLEM, NOT THE SYMPTOM: CARPAL TUNNEL CONUNDRUM

Often, we have people walk through our doors because they have been suffering with some chronic pain: carpal tunnel, elbow tendinitis, plantar fasciitis, low back discomfort, hip pain, etc. They learned from a friend, who had experienced the same symptoms, that we had helped them by developing a series of exercises to address their structure and pain symptoms. They ask if we could show them the exercises we gave their friend because they have the same pain. Our answer, without appearing rude or smug, is either "no," or "it depends." We then have to explain our answer.

Have you ever experienced a headache because you hit your head on the kitchen cabinet? Or, have you ever experienced a high level of stress and a headache appeared? Have you ever eaten ice cream too fast and suddenly a headache came on? Are you going to treat each of these headaches the same way? No, because the cause of each headache is different. The same can be said of symptoms like carpal tunnel syndrome. It is merely an uncomfortable signal that something is not quite right. Your body is moving in a way which creates pain, inflammation, irritation, etc.

The reason why the carpal tunnel symptoms appear could come from a myriad of reasons. Yes, repetitive movements can often cause pain and irritation. However, if the movement was the problem, then wouldn't everyone who performed the movement get carpal tunnel pain? Perhaps it would be more accurate to say that the body that performed the repetitive motion tried to organize the movement in a way which eventually brought on the symptoms. What if someone had sustained an injury in a completely different region of their body, which subconsciously forced them to reorganize the way their whole body moved? Could that have brought on carpal tunnel pain? Sound too far-fetched? Think about this scenario.

An active woman who works in a local grocery store as a cashier took her dog on a walk. She exercises daily and has never experienced any chronic pain or discomfort. During the walk her dog saw a squirrel and bolted after it. When it bolted, it pulled the woman to the ground. The woman twisted her ankle and severely bruised her left hip when she fell. When the dog eventually came back, she put him on the leash and limped home. During the walk home her body had to find the least painful way to move. It began to reorganize how each joint cooperated with one another to get her home.

The next day at work, she stood behind the register, reaching from right to left. As she scanned each grocery item, she could feel the left hip bruise and the slightly swollen ankle. Her body now had to subconsciously reorganize how she did her job in order to get away from the pain. She wasn't able to easily sway her hips side to side or bear as much weight on her injured ankle as she normally would. Instead she began to subtly shift her weight onto her right leg and reach more with her upper body and arms. That action caused her body to rotate over her right hip and allowed her left hip to drop just a little. With her pelvis tilted, her spine began to lean to the left, so the muscles along her back had to pull more to the right while her ribs tried to balance out the hip rotation by turning left. At the same time, she tried to lift her body weight off her left hip and ankle by lifting her shoulders a little higher. She had found a successful way to get the job done!

Unfortunately, over the next week, her new-found, successful way of getting the job done became the adapted way of working. Her body normalized this posture and how she moved since the fall. Even though the pain had gone away, her compensatory pattern of movement remained like a shadow of what had happened. Six months later the cashier began to notice tingling in her right hand and a loss of strength. She tried stretching and massaging the wrist and hand but it did not provide lasting relief. A few more months went by and she began to wear a wrist brace because pain was beginning to occur. A few months later she went on disability and considered surgery for her recently diagnosed "Carpal Tunnel." She talked to a friend who had found relief from his carpal tunnel pain by training with us and getting a series of centering exercises. When she came in asking for the exercises, what did we say? No, of course. It depends.

Her friend experienced carpal tunnel pain because he was mountain biking and broke his collarbone when he fell off his bike. His desk job and frequent mountain bike excursions forced him to organize the way his body moved in a completely different manner than the cashier. His reorganized movements brought on the same symptom, but the solution for her would not be the same, just as the treatment for the ice cream headache versus the headache caused by hitting your forehead on the kitchen cabinet would not be the same.

Instead of giving her the same exercises, we needed to be detectives and look for clues to the root cause of the symptoms. We began asking questions and eventually found out about the fall she had when her dog went after the squirrel and which had occurred a year ago. She didn't see the significance of the event and she couldn't make the connection with her carpal tunnel pain. Then we began asking her body questions. What if we were able to train the body to change the subconscious pattern of movement? What if we allowed the body to bear weight on the previously injured ankle and enabled the shoulders to relax and lower in a pain free environment (remember the reason she did it was because she was experiencing pain)?

Would you believe that her exercise program for her carpal tunnel did not involve isolated wrist exercises or stretches? The program involved creating better balance in her hip position and improving her ankle motion. It involved getting her to breathe properly and deeply to allow the body to experience shoulders lifting, lowering, and relaxing. In the program we also reorganized the way she walked, stood, reached, pushed, and pulled. It addressed the problem and suddenly the symptom diminished. Not long after performing the program, her pain was gone. She went back to work and began enjoying her life again.

APPENDIX
PROGRAM DESIGN CHART

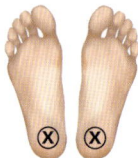
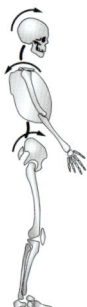

1

MISSING

Pelvic – Posterior Tilt
Rib – Anterior Tilt
Shoulder – Extension

	MOBILITY & FLEXIBILITY	STRENGTH MOVEMENTS	SOFT TISSUE WORK (SMR)
S T R U C T U R A L	Cervical Spine Matrix Foot Circles & Flexes Floor Cogs Gluteals Knee Circles Latissimus Dorsi Quadriceps Quadruped Cogs Sagittal Arm Cogs-split Stance Wall Cogs Wrist Circles	1-Arm Rotation - Forward 1-Arm Low Row 1-Arm Opposite Side Rotational Overhead Press Back Lunge Back Lunge W/ipsilateral Reach Back Lunge W/contralateral Reach Crossover Lunge W/contralateral Reach Crossover Step Up Front Lunge W/ipsilateral Reach Horizontal Press W/pronation (Bilateral) Lateral Lunge Lateral Lunge W/ipsilateral Oh Reach Lateral Lunge W/lateral Overhead Reach Away Lateral Lungew/lateral Overhead Reach Toward Lateral Step Up Shoulder Matrix Rotational Step Up Rotation Driving Across Single Leg Deadlift W/contralateral One Arm Row Split Squat W/ipsilateral Reach	Feet Forearms Hip Flexors Lower Back Mid-back Quadriceps Shoulders (Rear Part)) Tibialis Anterior (Shins) Triceps

	MOBILITY & FLEXIBILITY	STRENGTH MOVEMENTS	SOFT TISSUE WORK (SMR)
F U N C T I O N A L	Arm Circles Calves Crossed Knee Lift Downward Dog Elbow Touches Foot Circles & Flexes Hamstrings Sagittal Arm In Opposition Cogs Sagittal Plane Cogs Toe Drags Type Ii Spine Wall Cogs Wrist Circles	1-Arm Horizontal Row 1-Arm Horizontal Press W/supination 1-Arm Pulldown 1-Arm Rotation Backward 1-Arm Same Side Rotational Overhead Press 4-way Overhead Band Pull Cable Rotation - Pulling Back Crossover Lunge Front Lunge Horizontal Press With Supination (Bilateral) Lat Pulldown (Bilateral) Lateral Lunge Lateral Lunge W/contralateral Reach Plank Clock Rotation Pulling Back Shoulder Matrix Single Leg Deadlift Split Squat W/contralateral Overhead Reach Squat (Bilateral) Squat W/bilateral Pull	Abdominals Biceps Calves Forearms Feet Gluteals Hamstrings Neck Pectorals (Chest) Shoulders (Front Part) Suboccipital Muscles Tensor Fascia Latae Upper Trapezius

2

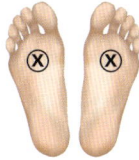

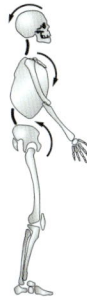

MISSING

Pelvic – Anterior Tilt
Rib – Posterior Tilt
Shoulder – Flexion

	MOBILITY & FLEXIBILITY	STRENGTH MOVEMENTS	SOFT TISSUE WORK (SMR)
S T R U C T U R A L	Arm Circles Calves Crossed Knee Lift Downward Dog Elbow Touches Foot Circles & Flexes Hamstrings Sagittal Arm In Opposition Cogs Sagittal Plane Cogs Toe Drags Type Ii Spine Wall Cogs Wrist Circles	1-Arm Horizontal Row 1-Arm Horizontal Press W/supination 1-Arm Pulldown 1-Arm Rotation Backward 1-Arm Same Side Rotational Overhead Press 4-way Overhead Band Pull Cable Rotation - Pulling Back Crossover Lunge Front Lunge Horizontal Press With Supination (Bilateral) Lat Pulldown (Bilateral) Lateral Lunge Lateral Lunge W/contralateral Reach Plank Clock Rotation Pulling Back Shoulder Matrix Single Leg Deadlift Split Squat W/contralateral Overhead Reach Squat (Bilateral) Squat W/bilateral Pull	Abdominals Biceps Calves Forearms Feet Gluteals Hamstrings Neck Pectorals (Chest) Shoulders (Front Part) Suboccipital Muscles Tensor Fascia Latae Upper Trapezius

	MOBILITY & FLEXIBILITY	STRENGTH MOVEMENTS	SOFT TISSUE WORK (SMR)
F U N C T I O N A L	Cervical Spine Matrix Foot Circles & Flexes Floor Cogs Gluteals Knee Circles Latissimus Dorsi Quadriceps Quadruped Cogs Sagittal Arm Cogs-split Stance Wall Cogs Wrist Circles	1-Arm Rotation - Forward 1-Arm Low Row 1-Arm Opposite Side Rotational Overhead Press Back Lunge Back Lunge W/ipsilateral Reach Back Lunge W/contralateral Reach Crossover Lunge W/contralateral Reach Crossover Step Up Front Lunge W/ipsilateral Reach Horizontal Press W/pronation (Bilateral) Lateral Lunge Lateral Lunge W/ipsilateral Oh Reach Lateral Lunge W/lateral Overhead Reach Away Lateral Lungew/lateral Overhead Reach Toward Lateral Step Up Shoulder Matrix Rotational Step Up Rotation Driving Across Single Leg Deadlift W/contralateral One Arm Row Split Squat W/ipsilateral Reach	Feet Forearms Hip Flexors Lower Back Mid-back Quadriceps Shoulders (Rear Part)) Tibialis Anterior (Shins) Triceps

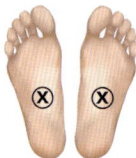

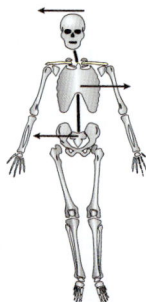

MISSING

Pelvic – Left Sway (Shift)

Rib – Right Lateral Flexion

Shoulder – R. Flexion
L. Abduction

STRUCTURAL

MOBILITY & FLEXIBILITY	STRENGTH MOVEMENTS	SOFT TISSUE WORK (SMR)
Ankle Tilts (Right Foot Bias) Arm Circles Cervical Spine Matrix Crossed Knee Lift (Right Side Bias) Downward Dog Floor Cogs Foot Circles & Flexes Frontal Plane Swaying Cogs Latissimus Dorsi Neck Glides Pectorals Quadriceps Quadruped Cogs Sagittal Arm Cogs Split Stance Type Ii Spine Wall Cogs	1-Arm Opposite Side Overhead Press (Right Arm Bias) 1-Arm Pulldown (Left Arm Bias) 1-Arm Straight Arm Pulldown (Left Arm Bias) 4-way Overhead Band Pull Back Lunge W/contralateral Reach (Left Leg Bias) Back Lunge W/ipsilateral Reach (Left Leg Bias) Diagonal Lunge (Right Leg Bias) Front Lunge W/contralateral Press (Right Leg Bias) Front Lunge W/ipsilateral Horizontal Press (Right Leg Bias) Front Lunge With Overhead Ipsilateral Press (Right Side Bias) Horizontal Press W/pronation (Left Arm/right Leg Bias) Lateral Lunge W/ipsilateral Reach (Right Leg Bias) Lateral Lunge W/ipsilateral Press (Right Leg Bias) Low-to-hi Press (Left Arm/right Leg Bias) Overhead Press (Right Arm Bias) Plank Clock Rotational Step Up (Right Leg Bias) Single Leg Deadlift (Right Leg Stance) Split Squat W/ipsilateral Overhead Press (Right Leg Forward) Straight Arm Pull (Left Arm Bias) Straight Leg Deadlift (Bilateral)	Feet Calves Left Abdominals Left Adductors Left Latissimus Dorsi Left Suboccipital Muscles Left Upper Trapezius Neck (Right Side Bias) Quadriceps Right Abductors Right Gluteals Right Mid-back Right Tensor Fascia Latae

FUNCTIONAL

MOBILITY & FLEXIBILITY	STRENGTH MOVEMENTS	SOFT TISSUE WORK (SMR)
Ankle Tilts (Left Foot Bias) Arm Circles Crossed Knee Lift (Left Side Bias) Downward Dog Foot Circles & Flexes Frontal Cogs Frontal Plane Swaying Cogs Gluteals Hamstrings Hip Circles (Right Leg Bias) Latissimus Dorsi Neck Glides Shift (Left Leg Fwd) Wall Cogs	1-Arm Opposite Side Overhead Press (Left Arm Bias) 1-Arm Straight Arm Pull (Right Arm Bias) 4-Way Overhead Band Pull Back Lunge W/contralateral Reach (Right Leg Bias) Back Lunge W/ipsilateral Reach (Right Leg Bias) Diagonal Lunge (Left Leg Bias) Front Lunge W/contralateral Press (Left Leg Bias) Front Lunge W/ipsilateral Horizontal Press (Left Leg Bias) Front Lunge With Overhead Ipsilateral Press (Left Side Bias) Horizontal Press W/pronation (Right Arm/left Leg Bias) Lat Pulldown (Right Arm Bias) Lateral Lunge W/ipsilateral Press (Left Leg Bias) Lateral Lunge W/ipsilateral Reach (Left Leg Bias) Lateral Step Up (Left Leg Bias) Low-to-hi Press (Right Arm/left Leg Bias) Overhead Press (Left Arm Bias) Plank Clock Rotational Step Up (Left Leg Bias) Single Leg Deadlift (Left Leg Stance) Split Squat W/ipsilateral Overhead Press (Left Leg Forward) Straight Leg Deadlift (Bilateral)	Feet Calves Left Abductors Left Gluteals Left Mid-back Left Tensor Fascia Latae Neck (Left Side Bias) Quadriceps Right Abdominals Right Adductors Right Latissimus Dorsi Right Suboccipital Muscles Right Upper Trapezius

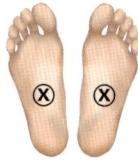
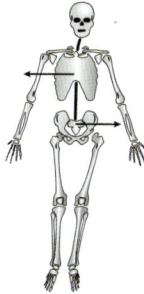

4

MISSING

Pelvic – Right Sway (Shift)

Rib – Left Lateral Flexion

Shoulder – L. Flexion
R. Abduction

STRUCTURAL

MOBILITY & FLEXIBILITY	STRENGTH MOVEMENTS	SOFT TISSUE WORK (SMR)
Ankle Tilts (Left Foot Bias)	1-Arm Opposite Side Overhead Press (Left Arm Bias)	Feet
Arm Circles	1-Arm Straight Arm Pull (Right Arm Bias)	Calves
Crossed Knee Lift (Left Side Bias)	4-Way Overhead Band Pull	Left Abductors
Downward Dog	Back Lunge W/contralateral Reach (Right Leg Bias)	Left Gluteals
Foot Circles & Flexes	Back Lunge W/ipsilateral Reach (Right Leg Bias)	Left Mid-back
Frontal Cogs	Diagonal Lunge (Left Leg Bias)	Left Tensor Fascia Latae
Frontal Plane Swaying Cogs	Front Lunge W/contralateral Press (Left Leg Bias)	Neck (Left Side Bias)
Gluteals	Front Lunge W/ipsilateral Horizontal Press (Left Leg Bias)	Quadriceps
Hamstrings	Front Lunge With Overhead Ipsilateral Press (Left Side Bias)	Right Abdominals
Hip Circles (Right Leg Bias)	Horizontal Press W/pronation (Right Arm/left Leg Bias)	Right Adductors
Latissimus Dorsi	Lat Pulldown (Right Arm Bias)	Right Latissimus Dorsi
Neck Glides	Lateral Lunge W/ipsilateral Press (Left Leg Bias)	Right Suboccipital Muscles
Shift (Left Leg Fwd)	Lateral Lunge W/ipsilateral Reach (Left Leg Bias)	Right Upper Trapezius
Wall Cogs	Lateral Step Up (Left Leg Bias)	
	Low-to-hi Press (Right Arm/left Leg Bias)	
	Overhead Press (Left Arm Bias)	
	Plank Clock	
	Rotational Step Up (Left Leg Bias)	
	Single Leg Deadlift (Left Leg Stance)	
	Split Squat W/ipsilateral Overhead Press (Left Leg Forward)	
	Straight Leg Deadlift (Bilateral)	

FUNCTIONAL

MOBILITY & FLEXIBILITY	STRENGTH MOVEMENTS	SOFT TISSUE WORK (SMR)
Ankle Tilts (Right Foot Bias)	1-Arm Opposite Side Overhead Press (Right Arm Bias)	Feet
Arm Circles	1-Arm Pulldown (Left Arm Bias)	Calves
Cervical Spine Matrix	1-Arm Straight Arm Pulldown (Left Arm Bias)	Left Abdominals
Crossed Knee Lift (Right Side Bias)	4-Way Overhead Band Pull	Left Adductors
Downward Dog	Back Lunge W/contralateral Reach (Left Leg Bias)	Left Latissimus Dorsi
Floor Cogs	Back Lunge W/ipsilateral Reach (Left Leg Bias)	Left Suboccipital Muscles
Foot Circles & Flexes	Diagonal Lunge (Right Leg Bias)	Left Upper Trapezius
Frontal Plane Swaying Cogs	Front Lunge W/contralateral Press (Right Leg Bias)	Neck (Right Side Bias)
Latissimus Dorsi	Front Lunge W/ipsilateral Horizontal Press (Right Leg Bias)	Quadriceps
Neck Glides	Front Lunge With Overhead Ipsilateral Press (Right Side Bias)	Right Abductors
Pectorals	Horizontal Press W/pronation (Left Arm/right Leg Bias)	Right Gluteals
Quadriceps	Lateral Lunge W/ipsilateral Reach (Right Leg Bias)	Right Mid-back
Quadruped Cogs	Lateral Lunge W/ipsilateral Press (Right Leg Bias)	Right Tensor Fascia Latae
Sagittal Arm Cogs Split Stance	Low-to-hi Press (Left Arm/right Leg Bias)	
Type Ii Spine	Overhead Press (Right Arm Bias)	
Wall Cogs	Plank Clock	
	Rotational Step Up (Right Leg Bias)	
	Single Leg Deadlift (Right Leg Stance)	
	Split Squat W/ipsilateral Overhead Press (Right Leg Forward)	
	Straight Arm Pull (Left Arm Bias)	
	Straight Leg Deadlift (Bilateral)	

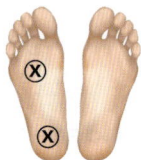

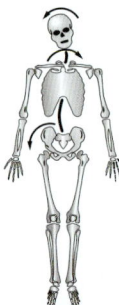

MISSING

Pelvic – Hike Right
Drop Left
Rib – Right Lateral Flexion
Shoulder – Left Abduction

5

STRUCTURAL

MOBILITY & FLEXIBILITY	STRENGTH MOVEMENTS	SOFT TISSUE WORK (SMR)
Ankle Tilts	1-Arm Opposite Side Overhead Press (Left Arm Bias)	Left Abdominals
Arm Circles	1-Arm Overhead Press - Opposite Leg Forward (Left Arm Bias)	Left Adductors
Arm Washrag	1-Arm Pulldown (Right Arm Bias)	Left Foot
Crossed Knee Lift	4-Way Overhead Band Pull	Left Gluteals
(Right Side Bias)	Back Lunge	Left Hamstrings
Crossover Twist	Back Lunge W/contralateral Reach (Left Leg Bias)	Left Mid-back
(Right Side Bias)	Cable Rotation - Driving Across (Right Bias)	Left Suboccipital Muscles
Elbow Touches	Crossover Lunge (Right Leg Bias)	Left Tensor Fascia Latae
Frontal Arm Cogs	Crossover Lunge W/contralateral Reach (Right Leg Bias)	Neck (Right Side Bias)
(Left Foot Fwd)	Crossover Step Up (Right Leg Bias)	Right Abductors
Frontal Plane Hiking Cogs	Crossover Step Up With Contralateral Overhead Reach (Right Leg Bias)	Right Biceps
Hamstrings	Front Lunge (Right Leg Bias)	Right Lats
Hip Circles (Left Leg Bias)	Front Lunge With Contralateral Horizontal Press (Right Leg Bias)	Right Quadriceps
Latissimus Dorsi	Front Lunge W/contralateral Overhead Press (Right Leg Bias)	Right Upper Trapezius
Neck Glides	Lateral Lunge (Right Leg Bias)	
Sagittal Arm Cogs	Lateral Lunge W/contralateral Reach (Right Leg Bias)	
Shift (Right Leg Fwd)	Lateral Lunge W/lateral Overhead Reach Away (Right Leg Bias)	
Transverse Cogs	Lateral Step Up (Right Leg Bias)	
Type Ii Spine Mobility	Rotational Lunge (Right Leg Bias)	
	Shoulder Matrix	
	Step Up (Right Leg Bias)	
	Step Up W/contralateral Overhead Press (Right Leg Bias)	

FUNCTIONAL

MOBILITY & FLEXIBILITY	STRENGTH MOVEMENTS	SOFT TISSUE WORK (SMR)
Ankle Tilts	1-Arm Opposite Side Overhead Press (Right Arm Bias)	Left Abductors
Arm Circles	1-Arm Overhead Press W/ Left Leg Fwd (Right Arm Bias)	Left Biceps
Arm Washrag	1-Arm Pulldown (Left Arm Bias)	Left Lats
Crossed Knee Lift	4-Way Overhead Band Pull	Left Quadriceps
(Left Side Bias)	Back Lunge	Left Upper Trapezius
Crossover Twist	Back Lunge W/contralateral Reach (Right Leg Bias)	Neck (Left Side Bias)
(Left Side Bias)	Cable Rotation Driving Across (Left Bias)	Right Abdominals
Elbow Touches	Crossover Lunge (Left Leg Bias)	Right Adductors
Frontal Arm Cogs	Crossover Lunge W/contralateral Reach (Left Leg Bias)	Right Foot
(Right Foot Fwd)	Crossover Step Up (Left Leg Bias)	Right Gluteals
Frontal Plane Hiking Cogs	Crossover Step Up With Contralateral Overhead Reach (Left Leg Bias)	Right Hamstrings
Floor Cogs	Front Lunge (Left Leg Bias)	Right Mid-back
Gluteals	Front Lunge With Contralateral Horizontal Press (Left Leg Bias)	Right Suboccipital Muscle
Neck Glides	Front Lunge W/contralateral Overhead Press (Left Leg Bias)	Right Tensor Fascia Latae
Quadriceps	Lateral Lunge (Left Leg Bias)	
Seated Hip Mobility	Lateral Lunge W/contralateral Reach (Left Leg Bias)	
Side Lying Arm Reach	Lateral Lunger W/lateral Overhead Reach Away (Left Leg Bias)	
Toe Drags	Rotational Lunge (Left Leg Bias)	
Transverse Arm Cogs	Shoulder Matrix	
	Step Up (Left Leg Bias)	
	Step Up W/contralateral Overhead Press (Left Leg Bias)	

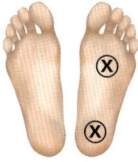

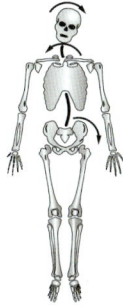

MISSING

Pelvic – Hike Left
Drop Right
Rib – Left Lateral Flexion
Shoulder – Right Abduction

	MOBILITY & FLEXIBILITY	STRENGTH MOVEMENTS	SOFT TISSUE WORK (SMR)
S T R U C T U R A L	Ankle Tilts Arm Circles Arm Washrag Crossed Knee Lift (Left Side Bias) Crossover Twist (Left Side Bias) Elbow Touches Frontal Arm Cogs (Right Foot Fwd) Frontal Plane Hiking Cogs Floor Cogs Gluteals Neck Glides Quadriceps Seated Hip Mobility Side Lying Arm Reach Toe Drags Transverse Arm Cogs	1-Arm Opposite Side Overhead Press (Right Arm Bias) 1-Arm Overhead Press W/ Left Leg Fwd (Right Arm Bias) 1-Arm Pulldown (Left Arm Bias) 4-Way Overhead Band Pull Back Lunge Back Lunge W/contralateral Reach (Right Leg Bias) Cable Rotation Driving Across (Left Bias) Crossover Lunge (Left Leg Bias) Crossover Lunge W/contralateral Reach (Left Leg Bias) Crossover Step Up (Left Leg Bias) Crossover Step Up With Contralateral Overhead Reach (Left Leg Bias) Front Lunge (Left Leg Bias) Front Lunge With Contralateral Horizontal Press (Left Leg Bias) Front Lunge W/contralateral Overhead Press (Left Leg Bias) Lateral Lunge (Left Leg Bias) Lateral Lunge W/contralateral Reach (Left Leg Bias) Lateral Lunger W/lateral Overhead Reach Away (Left Leg Bias) Rotational Lunge (Left Leg Bias) Shoulder Matrix Step Up (Left Leg Bias) Step Up W/contralateral Overhead Press (Left Leg Bias)	Left Abductors Left Biceps Left Lats Left Quadriceps Left Upper Trapezius Neck (Left Side Bias) Right Abdominals Right Adductors Right Foot Right Gluteals Right Hamstrings Right Mid-back Right Suboccipital Muscle Right Tensor Fascia Latae

	MOBILITY & FLEXIBILITY	STRENGTH MOVEMENTS	SOFT TISSUE WORK (SMR)
F U N C T I O N A L	Ankle Tilts Arm Circles Arm Washrag Crossed Knee Lift (Right Side Bias) Crossover Twist (Right Side Bias) Elbow Touches Frontal Arm Cogs (Left Foot Fwd) Frontal Plane Hiking Cogs Hamstrings Hip Circles (Left Leg Bias) Latissimus Dorsi Neck Glides Sagittal Arm Cogs Shift (Right Leg Fwd) Transverse Cogs Type Ii Spine Mobility	1-Arm Opposite Side Overhead Press (Left Arm Bias) 1-Arm Overhead Press - Opposite Leg Forward (Left Arm Bias) 1-Arm Pulldown (Right Arm Bias) 4-Way Overhead Band Pull Back Lunge Back Lunge W/contralateral Reach (Left Leg Bias) Cable Rotation - Driving Across (Right Bias) Crossover Lunge (Right Leg Bias) Crossover Lunge W/contralateral Reach (Right Leg Bias) Crossover Step Up (Right Leg Bias) Crossover Step Up With Contralateral Overhead Reach (Right Leg Bias) Front Lunge (Right Leg Bias) Front Lunge With Contralateral Horizontal Press (Right Leg Bias) Front Lunge W/contralateral Overhead Press (Right Leg Bias) Lateral Lunge (Right Leg Bias) Lateral Lunge W/contralateral Reach (Right Leg Bias) Lateral Lunge W/lateral Overhead Reach Away (Right Leg Bias) Lateral Step Up (Right Leg Bias) Rotational Lunge (Right Leg Bias) Shoulder Matrix Step Up (Right Leg Bias) Step Up W/contralateral Overhead Press (Right Leg Bias)	Left Abdominals Left Adductors Left Foot Left Gluteals Left Hamstrings Left Mid-back Left Suboccipital Muscles Left Tensor Fascia Latae Neck (Right Side Bias) Right Abductors Right Biceps Right Lats Right Quadriceps Right Upper Trapezius

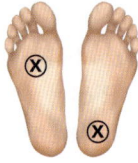
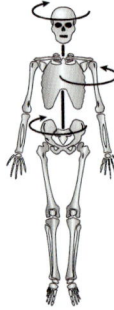

MISSING

Pelvic – Left Rotation
Rib – Right Rotation
Shoulder –
Left-Internal Rotation
Right-External Rotation

7

	MOBILITY & FLEXIBILITY	STRENGTH MOVEMENTS	SOFT TISSUE WORK (SMR)
S T R U C T U R A L	Alternating Sagittal Arm Cogs Ankle Tilts (Right Foot Bias) Arm Circles Arm Washrag Elbow Circles Knee Circles Latissimus Dorsi (Right Side Bias) Pectorals Seated Hip Mobility Side Lying Arm Reach T-spine Mobility In Quadruped Toe Drags Transverse Arm Cogs Transverse Cogs (Left Leg Fwd)	1-Arm Horizontal Press (Right Bias) 1-Arm Horizontal Row (Left Arm Bias) 1-Arm Low Row (Left Arm Bias) 1-Arm Opposite Rotational Overhead Press (Right Arm Bias) 1-Arm Pulldown (Right Arm Bias) 1-Arm Rotation Backward (Left Arm Bias) 1-Arm Same Side Overhead Press (Left Arm Bias) 1-Arm Straight Arm Pulldown (Left Arm Bias) Bent Over Row (Bilateral) Crossover Lunge (Left Bias) Crossover Step Up (Left Leg Bias) Crossover Step Up With Contralateral Overhead Reach (Left Leg Bias) Front Lunge (Left Leg Bias) Front Lunge W/contralateral Press (Left Leg Bias) Front Lunge W/ipsilateral Horizontal Press (Right Side Bias) Lat Pulldown (Bilateral) Pull Up (Bilateral) Push Up (Bilateral) Rotational Lunge (Left Leg Bias) Rotational Step Up (Left Leg Bias) Shoulder Matrix Shoulder Press (Bilateral) Single Leg Deadlift (Left Leg Bias) Single Leg Deadlift W/1-arm Low Row (Right Leg Bias) Split Squat (Left Leg Forward Bias) Split Squat W/rear Leg Raised (Left Leg Forward Bias)	Feet Forearms Left Abdominals Left Biceps Left Gluteals Left Lats Left Quadriceps Left Shoulder (Front Part) Left Tensor Fascia Latae Neck (Right Side Bias) Right Calf Right Hamstrings Right Hip Flexors Right Mid-back Right Occiput Right Pectorals Right Shoulder (Rear Part) Right Triceps

	MOBILITY & FLEXIBILITY	STRENGTH MOVEMENTS	SOFT TISSUE WORK (SMR)
F U N C T I O N A L	Alternating Sagittal Arm Cogs Ankle Tilts (Left Foot Bias) Arm Circles Arm Washrag Elbow Circles Latissimus Dorsi (Left Side Bias) Knee Circles Pectorals Seated Hip Mobility Side Lying Arm Reach T-spine Mobility In Quadruped Toe Drags Transverse Arm Cogs Transverse Cogs (Right Leg Fwd)	1-Arm Horizontal Press (Left Arm Bias) 1-Arm Horizontal Row (Right Arm Bias) 1-Arm Low Row (Right Arm Bias) 1-Arm Opposite Rotational Overhead Press (Left Arm Bias) 1-Arm Pulldown (Left Arm Bias) 1-Arm Rotation Backward (Right Arm Bias) 1-Arm Same Side Rotational Overhead Press (Right Arm Bias) 1-Arm Straight Arm Pulldown (Right Arm Bias) Bent Over Row (Bilateral) Crossover Lunge (Right Leg Bias) Crossover Step Up (Right Leg Bias) Crossover Step Up With Contralateral Overhead Reach (Right Leg Bias) Front Lunge W/contra Press (Right Leg Bias) Front Lunge W/ipsilateral Horizontal Press (Right Leg Bias) Lat Pulldown (Bilateral) Pull Up (Bilateral) Push Up (Bilateral) Rotational Lunge (Right Leg Bias) Rotational Step Up (Right Leg Bias) Shoulder Matrix Shoulder Press (Bilateral) Single Leg Deadlift (Right Leg Bias) Single Leg Deadlift W/1-arm Low Row (Right Leg Bias) Split Squat (Right Leg Forward Bias) Split Squat W/rear Leg Raised (Right Leg Forward Bias)	Feet Forearms Left Calf Left Hamstrings Left Hip Flexors Left Mid-back Left Occiput Left Pectorals Left Shoulder (Rear Part) Left Triceps Neck (Left Side Bias) Right Abdominals Right Biceps Right Gluteals Right Quadriceps Right Lats Right Shoulder (Front Part) Right Tensor Fascia Latae

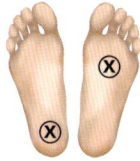 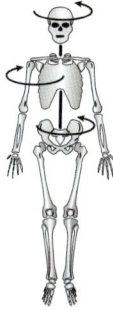

MISSING

Pelvic – Right Rotation
Rib – Left Rotation
Shoulder –
Left-External Rotation
Right-Internal Rotation

STRUCTURAL

MOBILITY & FLEXIBILITY	STRENGTH MOVEMENTS	SOFT TISSUE WORK (SMR)
Alternating Sagittal Arm Cogs Ankle Tilts (Left Foot Bias) Arm Circles Arm Washrag Elbow Circles Latissimus Dorsi (Left Side Bias) Knee Circles Pectorals Seated Hip Mobility Side Lying Arm Reach T-spine Mobility In Quadruped Toe Drags Transverse Arm Cogs Transverse Cogs (Right Leg Fwd)	1-Arm Horizontal Press (Left Arm Bias) 1-Arm Horizontal Row (Right Arm Bias) 1-Arm Low Row (Right Arm Bias) 1-Arm Opposite Rotational Overhead Press (Left Arm Bias) 1-Arm Pulldown (Left Arm Bias) 1-Arm Rotation Backward (Right Arm Bias) 1-Arm Same Side Rotational Overhead Press (Right Arm Bias) 1-Arm Straight Arm Pulldown (Right Arm Bias) Bent Over Row (Bilateral) Crossover Lunge (Right Leg Bias) Crossover Step Up (Right Leg Bias) Crossover Step Up With Contralateral Overhead Reach (Right Leg Bias) Front Lunge W/contra Press (Right Leg Bias) Front Lunge W/ipsilateral Horizontal Press (Right Leg Bias) Lat Pulldown (Bilateral) Pull Up (Bilateral) Push Up (Bilateral) Rotational Lunge (Right Leg Bias) Rotational Step Up (Right Leg Bias) Shoulder Matrix Shoulder Press (Bilateral) Single Leg Deadlift (Right Leg Bias) Single Leg Deadlift W/1-arm Low Row (Right Leg Bias) Split Squat (Right Leg Forward Bias) Split Squat W/rear Leg Raised (Right Leg Forward Bias)	Feet Forearms Left Calf Left Hamstrings Left Hip Flexors Left Mid-back Left Occiput Left Pectorals Left Shoulder (Rear Part) Left Triceps Neck (Left Side Bias) Right Abdominals Right Biceps Right Gluteals Right Quadriceps Right Lats Right Shoulder (Front Part) Right Tensor Fascia Latae

FUNCTIONAL

MOBILITY & FLEXIBILITY	STRENGTH MOVEMENTS	SOFT TISSUE WORK (SMR)
Alternating Sagittal Arm Cogs Ankle Tilts (Right Foot Bias) Arm Circles Arm Washrag Elbow Circles Knee Circles Latissimus Dorsi (Right Side Bias) Pectorals Seated Hip Mobility Side Lying Arm Reach T-spine Mobility In Quadruped Toe Drags Transverse Arm Cogs Transverse Cogs (Left Leg Fwd)	1-Arm Horizontal Press (Right Bias) 1-Arm Horizontal Row (Left Arm Bias) 1-Arm Low Row (Left Arm Bias) 1-Arm Opposite Rotational Overhead Press (Right Arm Bias) 1-Arm Pulldown (Right Arm Bias) 1-Arm Rotation Backward (Left Arm Bias) 1-Arm Same Side Overhead Press (Left Arm Bias) 1-Arm Straight Arm Pulldown (Left Arm Bias) Bent Over Row (Bilateral) Crossover Lunge (Left Leg Bias) Crossover Step Up (Left Leg Bias) Crossover Step Up With Contralateral Overhead Reach (Left Leg Bias) Front Lunge (Left Leg Bias) Front Lunge W/contralateral Press (Left Leg Bias) Front Lunge W/ipsilateral Horizontal Press (Right Side Bias) Lat Pulldown (Bilateral) Pull Up (Bilateral) Push Up (Bilateral) Rotational Lunge (Left Leg Bias) Rotational Step Up (Left Leg Bias) Shoulder Matrix Shoulder Press (Bilateral) Single Leg Deadlift (Left Leg Bias) Single Leg Deadlift W/1-arm Low Row (Right Leg Bias) Split Squat (Left Leg Forward Bias) Split Squat W/rear Leg Raised (Left Leg Forward Bias)	Feet Forearms Left Abdominals Left Biceps Left Gluteals Left Lats Left Quadriceps Left Shoulder (Front Part) Left Tensor Fascia Latae Neck (Right Side Bias) Right Calf Right Hamstrings Right Hip Flexors Right Mid-back Right Occiput Right Pectorals Right Shoulder (Rear Part) Right Triceps

ACKNOWLEDGMENTS

I would like to give deep thanks to my wife, Dana, for all the years of support and being my biggest cheerleader. Thanks to my long-time friend, surf companion, and principal photographer, Gary Irving, for another session of patience and insight. Thank you to the thousands of clients over the past quarter century; whether you knew it or not, you were my canvas on which we painted beautiful, changing landscapes. Thank you to the best staff of trainers anyone could hope for; your eagerness to learn propelled me to learn even more. Thank you to my colleagues Tom McCook, Bob McAtee, Wendy Willis, Helen Hall, Dave Hedges, and Michael Karim, who helped shape this book with their honest comments and questions during the peer review. Thank you to my mentors, Geoff Gluckman, Gary Ward, and Chris Sritharan. I do not claim to have ever had a unique thought at any time in my life. I am merely the messenger who shares what he has learned and will be forever grateful to all my teachers.

GLOSSARY

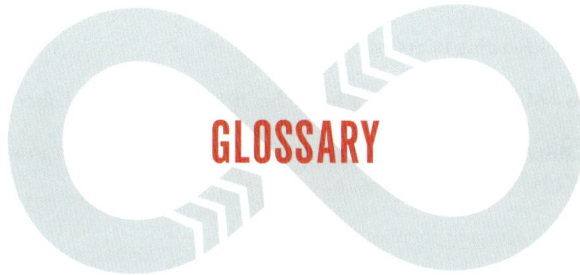

Abduction - The movement of a part of the body away from the midline of the body, or from another part.

Adduction - The moment of a part of the body toward the midline of the body, or toward another part.

Ambidextrous - The ability to use either left or right hand equally.

Arthrokinetic Reflex - The way in which joint motion can inhibit or activate muscles.

Asymmetry - Lack of equality or balance between parts.

Atrophy - A reduction or wasting away of body tissue as a result of the degeneration of cells.

Autonomic Nervous System (ANS) - The part of the nervous system responsible for the regulation of body functions not consciously controlled.

Base of Support - The area beneath a person that surrounds every point of contact the body makes against the ground.

Bilateral - Relating to both sides of the body.

Biomechanics - The laws pertaining to the movement of a body.

Center of Mass - The point representing the average mass in or around a body.

Cervical Spine - The seven vertebrae connecting the skull to the thoracic spine, that make up the neck.

Cogs - Two or more connected circular movements that move in opposing directions.

Compression - To reduce space between two points (muscle and soft tissue).

Concentric Contraction - The type of muscular contraction that causes the muscle to shorten.

Contralateral - Relating to opposing sides.

Dorsiflexion - Motion at the foot or hand that flexes in an upward direction.

Eccentric Contraction - The type of muscular contraction that causes the muscle to length.

Extension - The action of increasing a joint angle.

External Rotation - Rotation away from the center of the body.

Flexion - The action of decreasing a joint angle.

Frontal Plane - The vertical line that separates the anterior and posterior sides of the body.

Gait Cycle - The time and sequence of movements taken during locomotion when one foot strikes the ground until the next time the same foot strikes the ground.

Gait Phase - A point in time during the gait cycle.

Hyperextension - The point which a joint extends beyond it's proper anatomical end range.

Hypertrophy - The increase in size of muscle fiber.

Impingement - An impact at a joint when two bones converge and create inflammation or irritation to the surrounding tissue.

Internal Rotation - Rotation toward the center of the body.

Ipsilateral - Referring to the same side of the body.

Isometric Contraction - The activation of a muscle that causes zero change in length.

Lateral Flexion - The bending or leaning of a body part laterally.

Lumbar Spine - The five vertebrae of the lower back that connect the thoracic spine to the sacrum.

Metatarsal - The long bones of the forefoot that lie between the three cuneiform bones, the cuboid, and the phalanges of the toes.

Neural Map - The neural network of nerves throughout the body that allows stimuli to travel back and forth from the body to the brain.

Parasympathetic Response - Part of the Autonomic Nervous System that regulates muscle relaxation.

Peripheral Vision - The portion of vision outside of the focal area.

Plantarflexion - Motion at the foot or hand that flexes in an downward direction.

Pronation - The rotation of the hand, forearm, or foot downward or toward the midline.

Repetitions - The number of movements in a set.

Rotator Cuff - Four muscles (infraspinatus, supraspinatus, subscapularis, and teres minor) surrounding the shoulder that connect the humerus to the scapula and clavicle.

Sagittal Plane - The vertical line that separates the left from right side of the body.

Scoliosis - The lateral deviation of the spine from the midline.

Sets - The number of times a group of movements is attempted.

Soft Tissue - Tissues that connect, surround, and support structures and organs of the body.

Stretch-Shortening Reflex - An active lengthening of muscle followed immediately by a shortening of the same muscle.

Supination - The rotation of the hand, forearm, or foot upward or away from the midline.

Symmetry - The balance between two sides.

Sympathetic Response - Part of the Autonomic Nervous System the regulates an increase of muscle tension.

Tension - To increase space between two points (muscle and soft tissue).

Thoracic Spine - The twelve vertebrae connecting the cervical spine to the lumbar spine.

Transverse Plane - The horizontal line that separates the top and bottom.

Unilateral - Referring to one side.

Vestibular System - A collection of structures of the inner ear responsible for balance.

ABOUT THE AUTHOR

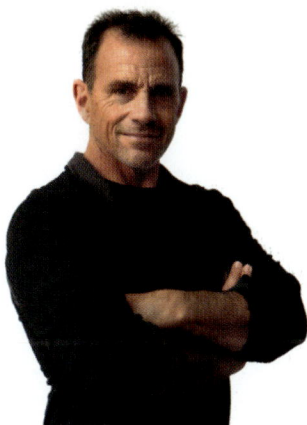

Rocky Snyder is a Certified Strength & Conditioning Specialist. He is a nationally recognized expert in human movement with nearly 30 years of professional experience and knowledge. Rocky has trained thousands of clients ranging from grandparents to professional athletes and Olympic champions. Aside from owning and operating his training studio in Santa Cruz, California, Rocky travels far and wide providing educational workshops to personal trainers, manual therapists, chiropractors, and physical therapists. He lives and surfs with his wife and two children in Aptos, California.